DERMATOLOGY - LABORATORY AND CLINICAL RESEARCH

NEW SKIN TOXICITIES FOR NEW ANTICANCER THERAPIES

DERMATOLOGY - LABORATORY AND CLINICAL RESEARCH

Additional books in this series can be found on Nova's website under the Series tab.

Additional e-books in this series can be found on Nova's website under the e-book tab.

DERMATOLOGY - LABORATORY AND CLINICAL RESEARCH

NEW SKIN TOXICITIES FOR NEW ANTICANCER THERAPIES

GIULIA GANZETTI
ANNA CAMPANATI
AND
ANNAMARIA OFFIDANI
EDITORS

NOVA BIOMEDICAL

New York

NOTICE TO THE READER

The Publisher has taken reasonable care in the preparation of this book, but makes no expressed or implied warranty of any kind and assumes no responsibility for any errors or omissions. No liability is assumed for incidental or consequential damages in connection with or arising out of information contained in this book. The Publisher shall not be liable for any special, consequential, or exemplary damages resulting, in whole or in part, from the readers' use of, or reliance upon, this material. Any parts of this book based on government reports are so indicated and copyright is claimed for those parts to the extent applicable to compilations of such works.

Independent verification should be sought for any data, advice or recommendations contained in this book. In addition, no responsibility is assumed by the publisher for any injury and/or damage to persons or property arising from any methods, products, instructions, ideas or otherwise contained in this publication.

This publication is designed to provide accurate and authoritative information with regard to the subject matter covered herein. It is sold with the clear understanding that the Publisher is not engaged in rendering legal or any other professional services. If legal or any other expert assistance is required, the services of a competent person should be sought. FROM A DECLARATION OF PARTICIPANTS JOINTLY ADOPTED BY A COMMITTEE OF THE AMERICAN BAR ASSOCIATION AND A COMMITTEE OF PUBLISHERS.

Additional color graphics may be available in the e-book version of this book.

Library of Congress Cataloging-in-Publication Data

ISBN: 978-1-63482-224-4
Library of Congress Control Number: 2015932295

Published by Nova Science Publishers, Inc. † New York

Contents

Preface

Targeted cancer therapies have revolutionized the therapeutic management of many neoplasms, modifying patients' prognosis and overall survival.

These drugs block the cancer's growth and spread by interfering with specific molecules which play a crucial role in the proliferation, differentiation and survival of cancer cells.

Targeted therapies act selectively on specific molecular targets related to cancers, whereas most of the conventional chemotherapies act on all rapidly dividing normal and neoplastic cells. Moreover, targeted therapies are often cytostatic and non-cytotoxic as standard chemotherapies. Taken together, these aspects appear important in reducing systemic toxicity and ensuring an improved safety profile.

The inhibition of epidermal growth factor receptor (EGFR), vascular growth factor (VEGF) and BRAF represents major achievements in research and development of solid tumors' epithelial therapy. This class of biologics is currently widely used in the treatment of metastatic and unresponsive neoplasms of the colon, pancreas, lung, (NSCLC), breast, head and neck and melanoma.

This book aims to emphasize skin toxicity associated with EGFR-, VEGF- and BRAF- inhibitors, focusing particularly on their clinical presentation, histopathological findings, and specific therapeutic options.

Chapter 1 - A better understanding of the role of epidermal growth factor receptor (EGFR), Vascular Endothelial Growth Factor (VEGF) and BRAF led to development of new cancer target therapies.

EGFRs represent a large family of tyrosine kinases (TKs) receptors over-expressed in several types of cancer, including breast, lung, oesophageal and head and neck cancer.

Two distinct therapeutic approaches are currently employed for targeting EGFR in cancer: on one hand the use of monoclonal antibodies and on the other hand the use of small molecules TK inhibitors (TKI).

VEGF and VEGF Receptors (VEGFR) act as potent stimulating agents in both physiological and pathological angiogenesis.

The central role of VEGF in tumor angiogenesis makes it an attractive target for anticancer therapy.

Anti-VEGF therapy inhibits the development of new tumor angiogenesis and promotes apoptosis of existing tumor blood vessels thereby intercepting the supply of oxygen and nutrition essential for tumor growth and metastasis.

Drugs targeting the VEGF pathways can be classified into four groups: anti-VEGF antibodies (Bevacizumab), soluble receptors binding directly to VEGF ligand (Aflibercept) and VEGFR TKI (Sorafenib, Sunitinib, Pazopanib).

Mitogen activated protein kinase (MAPK) cascade plays an important role in cellular proliferation and differentiation and contributes to the survival and growth of tumor cells. BRAF attends to transfer signals from activated cell surface growth factor receptors to numerous intracellular effectors, including transcription factors and regulators of apoptosis. BRAF selective inhibitors were developed for the treatment of metastatic malignant melanoma with V600 BRAF mutation. The two drugs in clinical use at this time are vemurafenib and dabrafenib.

Chapter 2 - The last few years have signed the introduction of EGFR inhibitors in the treatment of several types of cancers, as non-small cell lung cancer and head neck malignancies. This class of drugs comprises monoclonal antibodies (cetuximab, panitumumab) and tyrosine kinase inhibitors (erlotinib and gefitinib).

Although generally well tolerated, these targeted drugs are related to muco-cutaneous adverse reactions in a significant number of treated patients. Papulo-pustular rash, also known as acneiform rash, is the most frequent adverse event which considerably influences patient's quality of life. This skin effect appears to be directly linked to the inhibition of EGFR action, despite the exact pathophysiology remains elusive.

Actually, no standardized guidelines are available for the management of EGFR-inhibitors' skin toxicities. Although the permanent drug discontinuation is rare, management of EGFR inhibitors' related toxicities needs a multidisciplinary approach and represents a great challenge for dermatologists who face these clinical entities.

Chapter 3 - The inhibition of the vascular endothelial growth factor receptor (VEGFR) represent an important step in the treatment of many neoplasms.

As for EGFR inhibitors, VGFR inhibitors are associated with cutaneous adverse effects that tend to increase patient's morbidity and influence patient's quality of life.

The incidence of cutaneous adverse events varies considerably by drug.

This manuscript aims to emphasize the skin toxicity associated with VEGFR inhibitors, focusing particularly on clinical presentation, pathogenetic mechanism, and therapeutic options.

Chapter 4 - In the last two years, a new era in the treatment options for patients with metastatic cutaneous melanoma has come. Targeted therapies with the inhibitors of the RAS-RAF-MEK-ERK pathway (BRAF inhibitors) have substantially changed the therapeutic management of advanced melanoma. These agents are able to induce remarkable results for patients, but at the same time they have introduced a therapeutic challenge in the field of melanoma, owing to drug resistance and their clinical toxicity, which represent the two most discussed issues. For Dermatologists, the most intriguing "off target" effects of these target therapies are cutaneous adverse reactions. The therapeutic management of skin toxicities is mandatory to improve patients' outcome and quality of life. Moreover it puts dermatologists in a never ever thought position in the therapy of advanced melanoma. This manuscript reports the state of the art of skin toxicity associated with BRAF inhibitors, focusing particularly on clinical presentation, histopathological findings, and specific therapeutic options.

Chapter 5 - For the definition of toxicity in cancer patients receiving chemotherapy / radiotherapy, a special assessment scale has been established by the National Cancer Institute (NCI) and indicated by the acronym NCI-CTCAE (Common Terminology Criteria National Cancer Institute for Adverse Events) used for reporting adverse events. The latest versions are the NCI-CTCAE v.3 from the year 2006 and NCI-CTCAE v.4 proposed in 2009.

Any adverse event is described through a severity scale including 5 severity degrees: grade 1 (mild), grade 2 (moderate), grade 3 (severe), grade 4 (if the sign/symptom represents a threat to the life or determines disability) and grade 5 (if the adverse event appears to be the cause of death of the patient in treatment).

This evaluation scale has nevertheless proven to be unsuitable and unable to accurately describe dermatological adverse events and in particular the papulopustular rash. It should be stressed that this is an evaluation system designed to define the toxicity secondary to the use of traditional chemotherapy or radiotherapy, and therefore unable to best describe the events related adverse to new targeted therapies. Hence the need to propose and develop new grading able to outline and describe more fully the adverse events related EGFR-Is. In this regard, version NCI-CTCAE v.4 updated in 2009 has been introduced, but, however, for dermatologists, it is still not suitable for assessing the severity of the skin lesions and especially to monitor their evolution over time.

In: New Skin Toxicities … ISBN: 978-1-63482-224-4
Editors: Giulia Ganzetti et al.

Chapter 1

New Targeted Anticancer Therapies: Classification and Mechanism of Action

M. Caramanti, MD, F. Morgese, MD, A. Savini, MD and R. Berardi, MD*
Medical Oncology, Università Politecnica Marche, Italy

Abstract

A better understanding of the role of epidermal growth factor receptor (EGFR), Vascular Endothelial Growth Factor (VEGF) and BRAF led to development of new cancer target therapies.

EGFRs represent a large family of tyrosine kinases (TKs) receptors over-expressed in several types of cancer, including breast, lung, oesophageal and head and neck cancer.

Two distinct therapeutic approaches are currently employed for targeting EGFR in cancer: on one hand the use of monoclonal antibodies and on the other hand the use of small molecules TK inhibitors (TKI).

VEGF and VEGF Receptors (VEGFR) act as potent stimulating agents in both physiological and pathological angiogenesis.

The central role of VEGF in tumor angiogenesis makes it an attractive target for anticancer therapy.

* Corresponding author: r.berardi@univpm.it.

Anti-VEGF therapy inhibits the development of new tumor angiogenesis and promotes apoptosis of existing tumor blood vessels thereby intercepting the supply of oxygen and nutrition essential for tumor growth and metastasis.

Drugs targeting the VEGF pathways can be classified into four groups: anti-VEGF antibodies (Bevacizumab), soluble receptors binding directly to VEGF ligand (Aflibercept) and VEGFR TKI (Sorafenib, Sunitinib, Pazopanib).

Mitogen activated protein kinase (MAPK) cascade plays an important role in cellular proliferation and differentiation and contributes to the survival and growth of tumor cells. BRAF attends to transfer signals from activated cell surface growth factor receptors to numerous intracellular effectors, including transcription factors and regulators of apoptosis. BRAF selective inhibitors were developed for the treatment of metastatic malignant melanoma with V600 BRAF mutation. The two drugs in clinical use at this time are vemurafenib and dabrafenib.

Introduction

Due to the heterogeneous nature of cancer, personalised medicine is essential and therefore it is necessary to have a clear knowledge of the pathology and molecular mechanisms of a disease, as well as the associated clinical characteristics.

Epidermal growth factor (EGF), Vascular Endothelial Growth Factor (VEGF) and BRAF are involved in the cellular uncontrolled proliferation and they are considered relevant targets for different types of malignancies.

EGFR Targeted Therapies

A better understanding of the role of EGF receptor (EGFR) both in the pathogenesis and in the progression of cancer has led to a revolution in cancer treatment strategy in the last decade. In particular EGFR has shown to play a key role in the development and growth of tumor cells, since it is involved in numerous cellular responses including proliferation and apoptosis. EGFRs represent a large family of tyrosine kinases (TKs) receptors over-expressed in several types of cancer, including breast, lung, oesophageal and head and neck cancer. EGFR and its family members are the major contributors of a complex signaling cascade that modulates growth, differentiation, adhesion, migration and survival of cancer cells.

Due to their multidimensional role in cancer progression, EGFR and its family members have emerged as attractive candidates for anti-cancer therapy [1].

The ErbB family of receptors includes four known members namely ErbB1/EGFR/HER1 (in humans), ErbB2/HER2/Neu, ErbB3/HER3 and ErbB4/HER4 which are transmembrane glycoproteins with molecular weights ranging from 170 to185 KDa [2].

EGFR family members share a common domain arrangement comprised of a cysteine-rich extracellular domain, a transmembrane domain and an intracellular TK domain with several phosphorylation sites. The extracellular domains are subdivided into four domains (I-II-III and IV) (Figure 1).

EGFR gene can present several deletions, moreover several point mutations can occur in the TK domain [3].

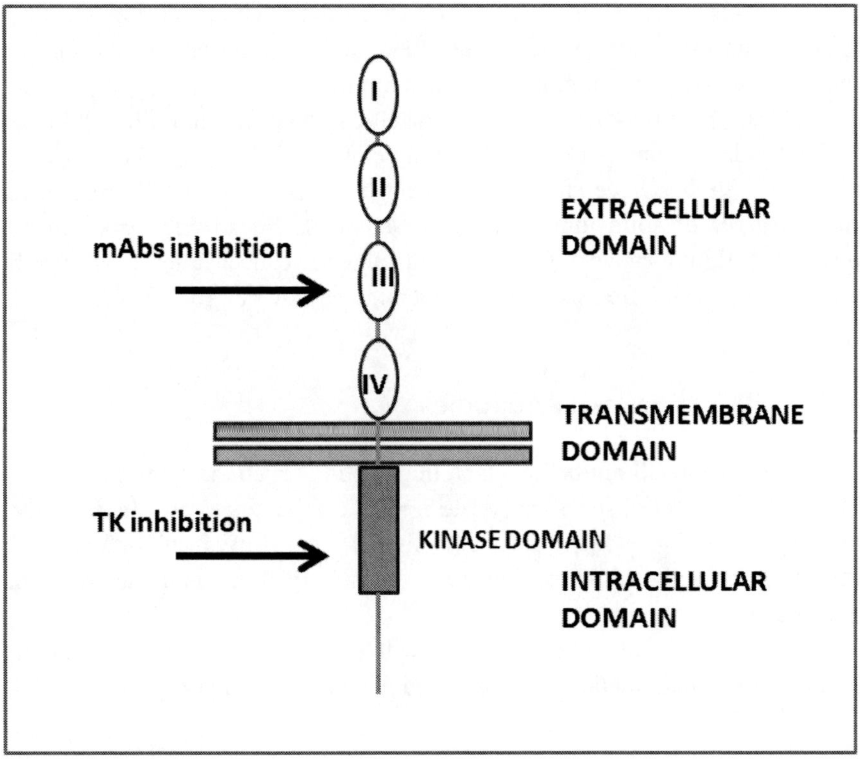

Figure 1.

EGFR may initiate cellular signaling cascades by itself through homodimerzation or through transactivation with other HER family members (heterodimerization).

ErbB family members can be activated by 13 known ligands, which include EGF, transforming growth factor alpha (TGF-α), amphiregulin (AR), betacellulin (BTC), heparinbinding EGF-like growth factor (HB-EGF), epiregulin (EPR), epigen (EPG) and neuregulins 1–6 (NRG) [4].

The receptor activation will further stimulate signaling cascades, which include the KRAS-BRAF-MEKERK pathway, phosphoinositide 3-kinase (PI3K), phospholipase C gamma protein pathway, the anti-apoptotic AKT kinase pathway and the STAT signaling pathway, which leads to cell proliferation, angiogenesis, migration, survival, and adhesion [5].

These cellular processes are often deregulated in malignant cells due to several mutations harbored in genes involved in these pathways.

Two distinct therapeutic approaches are currently employed for targeting EGFR in cancer: on one hand the use of monoclonal antibodies and on the other hand he use of small molecules TK inhibitors.

Anti-EGFR antibodies bind to extracellular domains and TK inhibitors target the ATP binding pockets in the intra-cellular TK domain (Figure 1).

Several studies have shown significant benefits of anti-EGFR agents in different types of solid tumors including colorectal, head and neck cancer, non-small cell lung cancer (NSCLC) and pancreatic cancer in terms of overall survival, progression free survival and overall response rate [6-10].

Anti-EGFR Monoclonal Antibodies

The monoclonal antibodies targeting EGFR, such as Cetuximab and Panitumumab, were specifically designed to be directed against the extracellular region which creates a ligand competitive inhibition, thus preventing receptor dimerization, auto-phosphorylation and downstream signaling [11].

These monoclonal antibodies also will induce receptor internalization, ubiqutinization, degradation and prolonged downregulation [12].

Cetuximab

Cetuximab is an approved human–murine chimeric anti-EGFR monoclonal antibody that binds to the second domain of EGFR thereby blocking its downstream signaling by prompting receptor internalization.

Increasing evidence shows that 60% of the patients expressing a KRAS wild-type tumor respond effectively to cetuximab treatment. This supported the use of KRAS as a biomarker in predicting tumor response in colorectal cancer [13].

Therefore Cetuximab was approved for the treatment of patients with KRAS wild type metastatic colorectal cancer both in monotherapy in patients who have failed with irinotecan-based chemotherapy or in combination with irinotecan or oxaliplatin-based therapy in the first line setting.

Moreover Cetuximab was approved by Food and Drug Administration (FDA) in 2004 and by European Medicines Agency (EMA) in 2008 in combination with platinum-based therapy for the treatment of metastatic squamous cell carcinoma of the head and neck and in combination with radiation therapy for locally advanced head and neck cancer.

Many head and neck squamous cell tumors do not show activity to EGFR targeting agents, as the response rate with such agents in monotherapy is consistently lower than 15% [14].

No predictive biomarker for head and neck squamous cell carcinoma has been found to date. Therapeutic resistance to anti-EGFR therapy may arise from mechanisms that can compensate for reduced EGFR signaling and/or mechanisms that can modulate EGFR-dependent signaling.

Panitumumab

Panitumumab is a totally human monoclonal antibody targeting EGFR.

Similarly to Cetuximab, colorectal cancer patients carrying the wild-type KRAS showed a promising response to panitumumab treatment [15].

Panitumumab was approved for the treatment of metastatic colorectal cancer in first line setting in combination with fluorouracil and oxaliplatin-based chemotherapy, or as a monotherapy in patients who have failed with irinotecan, oxaliplatin and fluorouracil-based chemotherapy.

However, not all patients experience a good response to anti-EGFR monoclonal antibodies, and given the risks for adverse effects associated with their use and their substantial cost, there is particular interest in identifying predictors of treatment benefit or lack thereof [16].

Genetic alterations may explain the resistance to anti-EGFR therapies [17].

In current clinical practice, KRAS mutation (codon 12 and 13) is mainly responsible for primary resistance to the EGFR target drugs, particularly cetuximab and panitumumab [18].

Thus the advantages of anti-EGFR monoclonal antibody treatment of colorectal cancer may be limited to KRAS wild-type patients [19].

EGFR Targeted Tyrosine Kinase Inhibitors

TK inhibitors (TKI) are small molecules that exist as adenosine triphosphate (ATP) analogues and inhibit EGFR signaling by competing and binding with ATP binding pockets on the intracellular catalytic kinase domain of receptor TKs, thereby preventing autophosphorylation and activation of several downstream signaling pathways [20].

They compete with ATP molecules that recognize the kinase active conformation. Irreversible inhibitors bind to the kinase active site covalently by specifically reacting with a nucleophilic cysteine residue. In addition, irreversible inhibitors have the advantage of prolonged clinical effects and a decreased need for frequent dosing, although it may compromise specificity and tolerability [21].

TKI such as erlotinib and gefitinib, have been approved for the treatment of NSCLC, showing an improvement in progression-free and overall survival, particularly in patients harboring activating EGFR mutations.

These activating mutations are more frequently observed in patients with adenocarcinoma histology, females, never smokers, and in those with Asian ethnicity [22,23].

The two most common EGFR mutations are short in-frame deletions of exon 19 and a point mutation (CTG to CGG) in exon 21 at nucleotide 257, resulting in the substitution of leucine by arginine at codon 858 (L858R) [24].

Gefitinib

Gefitinib is an oral reversible EGFR TKI belonging to the small molecule class (quinazoline-derivative molecule) [25]. It inhibits both autophosphorylation and downstream signaling, competing reversibly with ATP. Gefitinib is approved for the treatment of patients with locally advanced or metastatic NSCLC harboring activating EGFR mutations.

Erlotinib

Erlotinib is a low molecular weight, orally bioavailable inhibitor of EGFR and it was the first targeted agent approved for second- and third-line treatment of NSCLC unselected patients. Similarly to Gefitinib, Erlotinib is approved for the treatment of patients with locally advanced or metastatic NSCLC harboring activating EGFR mutations. Erlotinib is also approved for the treatment of locally advanced, unresectable or metastatic pancreatic cancer patients in combination with a gemcitabine [6, 10].

Unfortunately, all responders eventually develop resistance, most commonly because of the emergence of a gatekeeper mutation in the kinase domain, such as T790M in EGFR-mutated NSCLC [26] or amplification of mesenchymal–epithelial transition factor (c-Met) [27].

VEGF Targeted Therapy

Angiogenesis is a complex process that is closely controlled by factors that stimulate or inhibit the formation of new blood vessels. Tumor angiogenesis is known to be different from the physiological angiogenesis and it has been shown to lead to the development of abnormal vascular architecture, changes in interaction between endothelial cells and perivascular cells, increase vascular permeability. Blood supply through newly generated tumor blood vessels is considered essential for tumor growth. Proangiogenic gene expression is increased by physiologic stimuli, such as hypoxia. Oncogene activation or tumor suppressor mutation can also drive the balance in favor of proangiogenic factors, stimulating the development of new blood vessels in and around the tumor, thus allowing the tumor to expand, invade surrounding tissues, and metastasize [28, 29].

Anti-angiogenic therapy inhibits tumor angiogenesis and promotes apoptosis of existing tumor blood vessels, thereby blocking the supply of oxygen and nutrition essential for tumor growth and metastasis. It was also suggested that anti-angiogenic therapy effectively normalizes abnormal vascular permeability, and thereby decreases the interstitial pressure, which may improve delivery of concomitantly used chemotherapeutic agents to tumor cells.

VEGF and VEGF Receptors (VEGFR) act as one of the most potent stimulating agents in both physiological and pathological angiogenesis [30, 31].

Tumors produce a series of angiogenic factors including VEGF.

VEGF is a glycoprotein with a molecular weight of 34–46 kDa produced by normal cells and tumor cells. It serves as soluble ligand to VEGFR proteins on the surface of vascular endothelial cells as homodimers.

Expression of the VEGF-encoding gene is regulated by various factors and stimuli, including hypoxia, acidosis, hormones, cytokines and various signalling molecules.

When VEGF is secreted by these factors and binds to VEGF receptor (VEGFR), the VEGFR activation leads to survival of immature endothelial cells by abolition of apoptosis, growth/migration of vascular endothelial cells and promotion of capillary vascular permeability [32-34].

The VEGF family is divided into six members: VEGF-A, VEGF-B, VEGF-E which act specifically on vascular endothelial cells and VEGF-C, VEGF-D and placental growth factor (PlGF) which act on lymphatic vessel endothelial cells [35, 36].

VEGF-A is one of the most essential regulator of vasculogenesis, angiogenesis and differentiation of progenitor endothelial cells.

VEGF-B and PlGF also stimulate angiogenesis in normal tissues, but their activities are much weaker than those of VEGF-A [37].

However, an increase in PlGF has been reported to promote pathological angiogenesis in tumors and inflammatory lesions [38, 39].

VEGF members interact with cell membrane receptors (VEGFRs), which consist of three subtypes, VEGFR-1, VEGFR-2, and VEGFR-3, and are structurally related to platelet-derived growth factor receptors (PDGFR).

All VEGFRs subtypes possess seven immunoglobulin- like domains in the extracellular region and a TK domain in the intracellular region [40, 41].

VEGFR-1 and VEGFR-2 are expressed in vascular endothelial cells and hematopoietic stem cells but they have also been detected in some tumor cells while the expression of VEGFR-3 is largely restricted to lymphatic endothelial cells [42, 43].

VEGF members have different affinities for one of three VEGFR subtypes. VEGF-A activates VEGFR-1 and VEGFR-2, whereas VEGF-B and PlGF bind only to VEFGR-1.

Although VEGFR-1 binds VEGF-A with about 10- fold higher affinity than VEGFR-2, VEGFR-1 is poorly activated in response to VEGF-A that performes most of its biological activity binding VEGFR-2.

It was reported that VEGFR-1 is weakly involved in mediating the physiological angiogenic response to VEGF; however stimulation of VEGFR-1 seemed to indirectly induce tumor angiogenesis *via* activation of monocytes and macrophages and VEGFR- 1 signaling seemed to be implicated in tumor growth and metastasis [44, 45].

In fact monocytes and macrophages migrate into tumor and inflammatory lesions to produce VEGF-A, VEGF-C, and cytokines, leading to tumor angiogenesis and lymphoangiogenesis *via* VEGFR-2 and VEGFR-3 [46, 47].

VEGFR-2 seems to be predominantly responsible for responses of vascular endothelial cells to VEGF under both physiological and pathological conditions. The binding of VEGF to VEGFR2 promotes activation of signaling pathways involved in endothelial cell proliferation, migration and survival and enhances vascular permeability [48].

The signals generated from different VEGFRs are different.

The TK domains of VEGFR-1 and VEGFR-2 are divided by an insertion of a 65-97 hydrophobic region. This insert acts as an important recognition site for kinase substrates. The complex signaling from VEGFRs uses multiple factors to determine the biological responses to VEGF. The factors form a network of pathways with different crosstalk and overlapping functions, as well as distinct functions [49].

The central role of VEGF in tumor angiogenesis makes it an attractive target for anticancer therapy.

Anti-VEGF therapy inhibits the development of new tumor angiogenesis and promotes apoptosis of existing tumor blood vessels thereby intercepting the supply of oxygen and nutrition essential for tumor growth and metastasis.

Some authors also suggested that anti-VEGF therapy effectively normalizes abnormal vascular permeability, and thereby decreases the interstitial pressure; others advanced that these effects may improve delivery of concomitantly used chemotherapeutic agents to tumor cells [50-52].

VEGF-A and VEGFR-2 are currently the main targets for antiangiogenic therapy.

VEGF is considered an attractive therapeutic target because it circulates in the blood and acts directly on vascular endothelial cells, so drugs that target VEGF do not need to penetrate tumor tissue to inhibit tumor angiogenesis. Besides VEGF acts on endothelial cells, which may be less likely to mutate to a treatment-resistant phenotype than genetically unstable tumor cells and they may be a more attractive target than tumor cells for long-term therapy [53].

Inhibitors of VEGF mediated angiogenesis have shown clinically meaningful survival benefits, both as monotherapy or in combination with chemotherapy, in clinical trials with different types of solid tumors [54, 55].

Drugs targeting the VEGF pathways can be classified into four groups:

1. anti-VEGF antibodies;
2. soluble receptors binding directly to VEGF ligand;
3. anti-VEGFR antibodies;
4. VEGFR TKI.

Bevacizumab

Bevacizumab is a recombinant humanized monoclonal antibody against VEGF-A, and inhibits the binding between VEGF-A and VEGFR resulting in the prevention of VEGFR activation and the subsequent signaling cascades.

It was approved:

- as first-line treatment for metastatic colorectal cancer in combination with chemotherapy;
- as first-line treatment of patients with unresectable locally advanced, recurrent or metastatic, non-squamous, NSCLC in combination with chemotherapy;
- as a single agent for patients with recurrent glioblastoma with progressive disease following prior therapy;
- in combination with paclitaxel as first-line treatment in patients with metastatic HER2-negative breast cancer;
- as first-line therapy in metastatic renal cell carcinoma in combination with interferon;
- as first-line therapy in combination with carboplatin and paclitaxel in advanced ovarian cancer [56-63].

Aflibercept

Aflibercept is a soluble fusion protein of the extracelluar domain of human VEGFR-1 and VEGFR-2 and the Fc region of IgG, designed to bind to VEGF in the circulating blood.

Aflibercept was approved, in combination with fluorouracil and irinotecan, for treatment of patients with metastatic colorectal cancer, resistant to oxaliplatin.

Aflibercept prevents VEGFR activation and downstream signaling because it efficiently binds VEGF-A and PlGF with high affinity.

Most prominent grade 3/4 toxicities reported in different studies with Aflibercept include proteinuria, hypertension, fatigue and headache [64].

Sunitinib

Sunitinib is an orally small-molecule multitarget type TKI targeting VEGFR1, VEGFR2, and VEGFR3 as well as Flt-3, PDGFR-a, PDGFR-h, and c-Kit.

Sunitinib is used for the treatment of renal carcinoma and gastrointestinal stromal tumors (GIST) [65-70].

Sorafenib

Sorafenib is a TKI inhibiting VEFGR-2, VEGFR-3, Raf kinase and extracellular signal-regulated kinases.

Sorafenib has been approved for advanced–stage renal cell carcinoma and for advanced-stage hepatocellular carcinoma (HCC) [71-77].

Pazopanib

Pazopanib is an oral TKI of VEGFR2. Pazopanib has been approved as first line in patients with metastatic renal cell carcinoma and in patients with relapsed or refractory advanced soft tissue sarcoma.

The most common adverse effects due to pazopanib are diarrhea, hypertension, hair color change, nausea, anorexia and vomiting. Elevation of alanine-leucine transaminase (ALT) was the most common laboratory abnormality [78-80].

BRAF Targeted Therapies

Mitogen activated protein kinase (MAPK) cascade plays an important role in cellular proliferation and differentiation and contributes to the survival and growth of tumor cells [81].

A small GTP binding protein (rat sarcoma: RAS), put on cell membranes, is actioned upon upstream activation of receptor TK by growth factors. RAS activation trigger intracellular signaling through wild-type RAF isoforms (including BRAF, CRAF, ERK and ARAF). These RAF isoforms produce homodimers and heterodimers in different combinations (e.g., BRAF: BRAF, BRAF: CRAF, etc.). These dimer complexes then lead to activation of MEK1 or MEK2, with subsequent signaling through activation of the ERK and MAPK pathways. ERK moves into the nucleus and animates progrowth signals [82].

In contrast, unregulated activation of the MAPK pathway can therefore conduct to malignancy.

As a component of the MAPK pathway, BRAF attends to transfer signals from activated cell surface growth factor receptors to numerous intracellular effectors, including transcription factors and regulators of apoptosis. It regulates the cell cycle entry through control of cyclin D1 expression and the suppression of p27KIP [83].

Then mutated BRAF exists as a monomer and it signals in constitutive fashion independent of upstream activation by receptor tyrosine kinase and RAS.

For their role in oncogenesis, the RAF protein kinases have been extensively studied.

In particular, BRAF mutations have been found in 10%–15% of colorectal carcinomas, 3% of lung adenocarcinomas and breast cancers, 20%–50% of serous ovarian cancers and 29%–69% of papillary thyroid cancers, 30-60% of melanomas and most recently hairy-cell leukemia, in all accounting for 7% to 8% of all cancers [84-94].

In each tumor type, the presence of a BRAF mutation has been correlated with a more aggressive disease and a worse prognosis.

In melanoma, the BRAF mutation in the primary lesion has not been shown to impact on disease-free interval or overall survival [95-97].

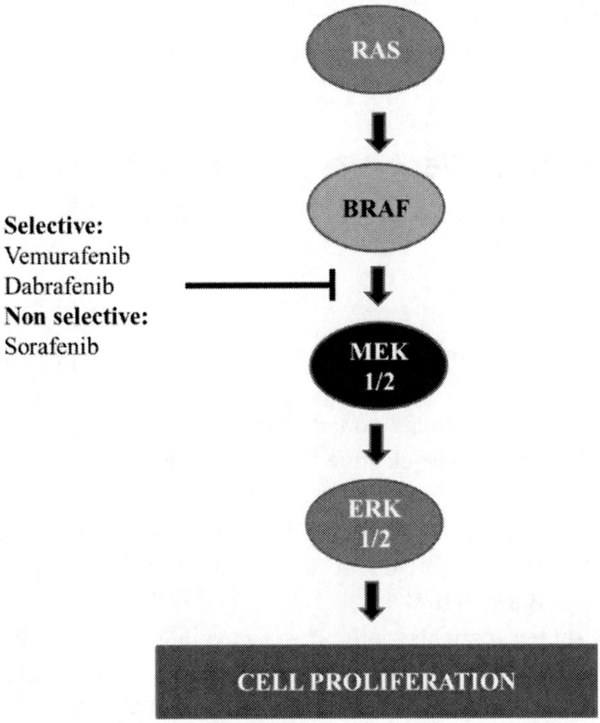

Figure 2.

However, after the development of metastatic melanoma, the median survival of patients with BRAF mutations has been characterized as shorter relative to patients with wild-type BRAF tumors [98-100].

BRAF mutations have been shown at exon 11 or exon 15 within the kinase domain. Approximately 80% of mutations derived from a single point mutation at amino-acid position 599 (now known as 600), which resulted in the substitution of a glutamic acid (E) for valine (V), V600E. Other substitutions include valine by lysine (V600K) (about 20%) and valine by arginine (V600R) (3% of all mutations).

Then the knowledge of the mutational landscape of melanoma disease clearly shows that the different clinical manifestations of melanoma also contrast in their molecular changes, which subsequently will be of importance for therapies directed against tumors bearing a distinct mutation [101-104].

Two types of BRAF inhibitors have been developed and tested in advanced melanoma: type 1 BRAF inhibitors that bind and arrest the active conformation of the BRAF kinase and type 2 BRAF inhibitors that bind to the inactive conformation of the kinase (Figure 2) [105].

Non-Selective BRAF Inhibitors (Type 2-Binding Mode)

Sorafenib

Sorafenib stabilises the enzyme with the DFG-loop flipped out of the ATP pocket [106].

It was the first drug studied to target the BRAF-mutated melanomas and it was initially developed as a selective CRAF, BRAFwt, and BRAFmut proteins inhibitor, with little selectivity for one isoform over another, but it was later found to have an inhibitory effect on other protein kinases as well, such as VEGF receptors 2 and 3, PDGF receptor, Flt-3, c-kit, FGF receptor 1, p38 MAPK, FMA, and RET [107].

In initial studies, patients were not selected on the basis of genotype. Due to sorafenib poor selectivity for the active conformation of BRAF induced by the V600E mutation, coupled with significant "off-target" activity, results were discouraged.

One potential explanation is that sorafenib has a higher affinity for other RAF isoforms as well as other pathways, thereby limiting its on target effects [108-115].

To date, no studies have detected any correlation between BRAF genotype (mutant versus wild-type) and response to sorafenib, either as a single agent or in combination with chemotherapy.

Selective BRAF Inhibitors (Type 1-Binding Mode)

The most promising results in patients with BRAF-mutated melanoma have been seen with drugs designed to selectively target the mutated and activated form of the BRAF kinase.

Type 1 inhibitors bind the active configuration of the kinase, stabilising the enzyme with the DFG-loop in the ATP pocket, inhibiting BRAF kinase and MAPK activity [116].

The two drugs in clinical use at this time are vemurafenib and dabrafenib.

Targeted inhibition of this signaling cascade translates into meaningful clinical benefit for patients with metastatic melanoma.

Vemurafenib

The first selective BRAF inhibitor to be developed in the clinical setting was vemurafenib [117-119].

Vemurafenib is orally administered ATP-competitive RAF inhibitors (wt BRAF IC50 100nM, mutated BRAF 31nM) and CRAF (IC50 48 nM) [120].

The BRAF-inhibitor vemurafenib in clinical trials, when delivered at the maximum-tolerated dose, induces strong inhibition of downstream signaling as determined by inhibition of pERK, reduction in Ki67 and inhibition of glucose uptake into melanoma metastases as measured by FDG-PET.

The median estimate half-life for vemurafenib is 57 hours. The apparent clearance of vemurafenib in patients with mild and moderate hepatic or renal impairment was similar to that in patients with normal hepatic or renal function respectively. In vitro studies have demonstrated that vemurafenib is a CYPP450 substrate [121].

Treatment with vemurafenib led to tumor regression in most patients with the BRAF V600E mutation, as well as improvements in PFS and OS [122-126].

Vemurafenib was approved by FDA in 2011 and by EMA in 2012 for the treatment of not-resectable or recurrent or metastatic melanoma (stage III and IV) positive for the BRAF V600 mutation that shows progressive disease. It especially benefits patients with increased LDH and patients in stage M1C who generally have a poor prognosis [127].

Dabrafenib

Another selective BRAF inhibitor is dabrafenib, an ATP-competitive inhibitor of BRAF V600E/D/K, wild-type BRAF and CRAF [128, 129].

Dabrafenib has less potency for inhibition of CRAF if it compared with vemurafenib. It has similar potency for inhibition of BRAFV600E and BRAFV600K.

In preclinical studies, dabrafenib inhibits the MAPK pathway in BRAFV600E melanoma cells, leading to decreased proliferation and regression in xenograft mouse models [130].

Dabrafenib has a median terminal half-life of approximately 8 hours after a single dose, with plasma concentrations peaking at a median of 2 hours and declining thereafter.

Dabrafenib metabolism is predominantly hepatic, with preclinical studies suggesting that the CYPP450 superfamily of mono-oxygenases plays a major role. The major route of excretion of dabrafenib in humans is fecal (70%), while renal excretion accounts for less than 20%.

Dabrafenib was approved by FDA in 2013 and by EMA in 2014 and it has the same therapeutic indication of Vemurafenib.

Resistance

Preliminary studies have already shown that a small number of patients develop primary resistance while others developed secondary resistance after an initial treatment response [131-133].

Multiple laboratory and clinical reports have started to detail mechanisms of both primary and acquired resistance to BRAFV600E inhibition in malignant melanoma [134-137].

The molecular biology of mutant RAF signaling is complex and significant efforts have been made to elucidate it.

Monitoring of MEK and ERK activation revealed distinct mechanisms of resistance, with elevated downstream phosphorylation in the setting of BRAF inhibition suggesting alternative MAPK pathway activation. Although multiple mechanisms appear to account for continued downstream signaling, utilization of different RAF isoforms, i.e, ARAF or CRAF, to circumvent BRAF inhibition has been identified. Specifically, developments of activating mutations of N-RAS kinase proteins, which tend to phosphorylate CRAF instead of BRAF, continue uncontrolled MAPK signaling. Another mechanism of resistance is acquisition of alternative splicing of BRAF (p61 BRAF), resulting in dimerization of RAF kinase and continued downstream ERK phosphorylation in the presence of RAF inhibitors. In addition, RAF-independent mechanisms have been identified with increased COT, a different serine/threonine MAP kinase, driving persistent MAPK cascade activation in the presence of BRAF inhibition. Alternatively, upregulation of receptor tyrosine kinases, such as platelet-derived growth factor receptor-β and insulin-like growth factor-1 receptor, confirms acquired MAPK-independent resistance [138-142].

Table 1. Principal anti-EGFR, VEGF and BRAF targeted therapies

DRUG	TARGET	TREATMENT INDICATIONS
Cetuximab	Anti-EGFR monoclonal antibody	• KRAS wild type metastatic colorectal cancer • metastatic squamous cell carcinoma of the head and neck
Panitumumab	Anti-EGFR monoclonal antibody	• KRAS wild type metastatic colorectal cancer
Gefitinib	EGFR TK inhibitor	• advanced or metastatic NSCLC with EGFR mutations
Erlotinib	EGFR TK inhibitor	• advanced or metastatic NSCLC • locally advanced unresectable or metastatic pancreatic cancer
Bevacizumab	Anti-VEGF monoclonal antibody	• metastatic colorectal cancer • non-squamous NSCLC • recurrent glioblastoma • metastatic breast cancer • metastatic renal cell carcinoma • - advanced ovarian cancer
Aflibercept	Soluble fusion protein anti VEGF	• metastatic colorectal cancer
Sunitinib	VEGFR TK inhibitor	• renal carcinoma • gastrointestinal stromal tumors (GIST)
Sorafenib	VEGFR TK inhibitor	• metastatic renal cell carcinoma • advanced-stage hepatocellular carcinoma
Pazopanib	VEGFR TK inhibitor	• metastatic renal cell carcinoma • relapsed or refractory advanced soft tissue sarcoma.
Dabrafenib	BRAF inhibitor	• not-resectable or recurrent or metastatic melanoma expressing BRAF V600 mutation
Vemurafenib	BRAF inhibitor	• not-resectable or recurrent or metastatic melanoma with BRAF V600 mutation

Recent preclinical studies have demonstrated that amplification of cyclin D1 (in up to 17% of BRAF V600E mutant melanomas) or loss of the tumor suppressor RB together with loss of the tumor suppressor phosphatase and tensin homolog (PTEN) may both contribute to intrinsic BRAF inhibitor resistance [143-145].

In the case of PTEN loss, BRAF inhibition was found to paradoxically activate AKT which prevented cell death by suppressing the levels of the pro-apoptotic protein BIM 94 [146, 147].

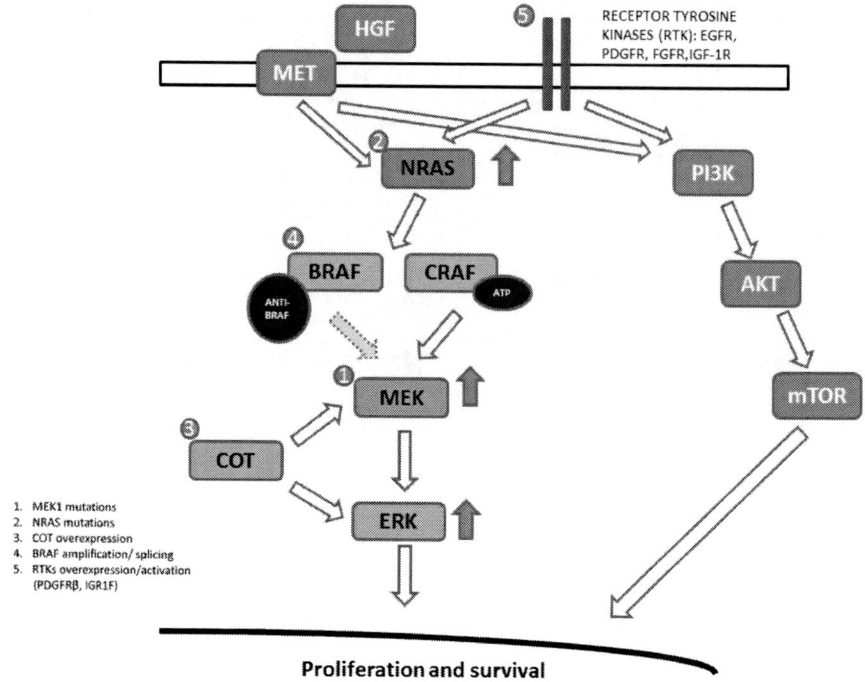

Figure 3.

The outcomes for patients with BRAF-mutant melanoma after development of resistance to BRAF targeting are poor.

Disease progression is observed in about 50% of patients receiving monotherapy within 6 months of treatment initiation [148].

Researchers who work to combine therapies to block multiple activated pathways in melanoma may overcome the intrinsic and acquired resistance to BRAF inhibitors. Given that the reactivation of the MAPK pathway is responsible for the majority of resistance, it is logical to combine BRAF inhibitors with MEK inhibitors (Figure 3) [149].

Conclusion

A growing number of new target therapies are being used in the treatment of cancer (table 1), also in combination with chemotherapy. These agents are generally well tolerated, but they may be accompanied by new distinct adverse effects, that may have a deep impact on the quality of life. Among these adverse events, in particular the skin toxicities were extensively studied.

References

[1] Grandis, JR; Sok, JC. Signaling through the epidermal growth factor receptor during the development of malignancy. *Pharmacol Ther.*, 2004, 102, 37–46.

[2] Olayioye, MA; Neve, RM; Lane, HA; et al. The ErbB signaling network: receptor heterodimerization in development and cancer. *EMBO J.*, 2000, 19, 3159–67.

[3] Kuan, CT; Wikstrand, CJ; Bigner, DD. EGF mutant receptor vIII as a molecular target in cancer therapy. *Endocr Relat Cancer.*, 2001, 8, 83–96.

[4] Yarden, Y; Sliwkowski, MX. Untangling the ErbB signaling network. Nat Rev Mol Cell Biol. 2001, 2, 127–37. **(11). Citri, A; Yarden, Y. EGF-ERBB signalling: towards the systems level. *Nat Rev Mol Cell Biol.* 2006, 7, 505–16.

[5] Baselga, J; Albanell, J. Epithelial growth factor receptor interacting agents. *Hematol Oncol Clin North Am.*, 2002, 16, 1041–63.

[6] Bareschino, MA; Schettino, C; Troiani, T; et al. Erlotinib in cancer treatment. *Ann Oncol.*, 2007, 18 (Suppl 6), vi35–41. vi35–vi41.

[7] Giaccone, G; Gonzalez-Larriba, JL; van Oosterom, AT; et al. Combination therapy with gefitinib;an epidermal growth factor receptor tyrosine kinase inhibitor; gemcitabine and cisplatin in patients with advanced solid tumors. *Ann Oncol.*, 2004, 15, 831–8.

[8] Petrelli, F; Borgonovo, K; Cabiddu, M; et al. Cetuximab and panitumumab in KRAS wild-type colorectal cancer: a meta-analysis. *Int J Colorectal Dis.*, 2011, 26, 823–33.

[9] Petrelli, F; Barni, S. Anti-EGFR-targeting agents in recurrent or metastatic head and neck carcinoma: A meta-analysis. *Head Neck.*, 2011, 10

[10] Rocha-Lima, CM; Soares, HP; Raez, LE; et al. EGFR targeting of solid tumors. *Cancer Control.*, 2007, 14, 295–304.

[11] Burgess, AW; Cho, HS; Eigenbrot, C; et al. An open-and-shut case? Recent insights into the activation of EGF/ErbB receptors. *Mol Cell.* 2003, 12, 541–52

[12] Sunada, H; Magun, BE; Mendelsohn, J; et al. Monoclonal antibody against epidermal growth factor receptor is internalized without stimulating receptor phosphorylation. *Proc Natl Acad Sci U S A.*, 1986, 83, 3825–9

[13] Van Krieken, JH; Jung, A; Kirchner, T; et al. KRAS mutation testing for predicting response toanti-EGFR therapy for colorectal carcinoma: proposal for an European quality assurance program. *Virchows Arch.*, 2008, 453, 417–31.

[14] Vermorken, JB; Herbst, RS; Leon, X; et al. Overview of the efficacy of cetuximab in recurrent and/or metastatic squamous cell carcinoma of the head and neck in patients who previously failed platinum-based therapies. *Cancer*, 2008, 112, 2710–2719.

[15] Hecht, JR; Patnaik, A; Berlin, J; et al. Panitumumab monotherapy in patients with previously treated metastatic colorectal cancer. *Cancer.*, 2007, 110, 980–8.

[16] Dahabreh, IJ; Terasawa, T; Castaldi, PJ; Trikalinos, TA. Systematic review: Anti-epidermal growth factor receptor treatment effect modification by KRAS mutations in advanced colorectal cancer. *Ann Intern Med*, 2011, 154, 37-49.

[17] Shackelford, RE; Whitling, NA; McNab, P; Japa, S; Coppola, D. KRAS Testing: A Tool for the Implementation of Personalized Medicine. *Genes Cancer*, 2012, 3, 459-466.

[18] Misale, S; Yaeger, R; Hobor, S; et al. Emergence of KRAS mutations and acquired resistance to anti-EGFR therapy in colorectal cancer. *Nature*, 2012, 486, 532-536.

[19] Cartwright, TH. Treatment decisions after diagnosis of metastatic colorectal cancer. *Clin Colorectal Cancer*, 2012, 11, 155-166.

[20] Ciardiello, F. Epidermal growth factor receptor tyrosine kinase inhibitors as anticancer agents. *Drugs.*, 2000, 60 (Suppl 1), 25–32.

[21] Slichenmyer, WJ; Fry, DW. Anticancer therapy targeting the erbB family of receptor tyrosine kinases. *Semin Oncol.*, 2001, 28, 67–79.

[22] Sun, S; Schiller, JH; Gazdar, AF. Lung cancer in never smokers – a different disease. Nat Rev *Cancer.*, 2007, 7 (10), 778–790.

[23] Subramanian, J; Govindan, R. Lung cancer in never smokers: a review. *J Clin Oncol.*, 2007, 25 (5), 561–570.

[24] Ladanyi, M; Pao, W. Lung adenocarcinoma: guiding EGFR-targeted therapy and beyond. *Mod Pathol.*, 2008, 21(Suppl 2), S16–S22.

[25] Baselga, J; Averbuch, SD. ZD 1839 ("Iressa") as an anticancer agent. *Drugs.*, 2000, 60 (Suppl 1), 33–40.

[26] Pao, W; Chmielecki, J. Rational; biologically based treatment of EGFR-mutant non-small-cell lung cancer. *Nat Rev Cancer.*, 2010, 10 (11), 760–774.

[27] Engelman, JA; Zejnullahu, K; Mitsudomi, T; et al. MET amplification leads to gefitinib resistance in lung cancer by activating ERBB3 signaling. *Science.*, 2007, 316 (5827), 1039–1043.

[28] Folkman, J. The role of angiogenesis in tumor growth. *Semin Cancer Biol*, 2002, 3, 65^71.

[29] Kerbel, RS; Folkman, J. Clinical translation of angiogenesis inhibitors. Nat Rev *Cancer*, 2002, 2, 727^39.

[30] Folkman, J. Tumor angiogenesis: therapeutic implications. *N Engl J Med.*, 1971, 285(21), 1182-6.

[31] Hanahan, D; Folkman, J. Patterns and emerging mechanisms of the angiogenic switch during tumorigenesis. *Cell.*, 1996, 86 (3), 353-64.

[32] Benjamin, LE. Tumorigenesis and the angiogenic switch. *Nat Rev Cancer*, 2003, 3, 401–10.

[33] Ferrara, N; Davis-Smyth, T. The biology of vascular endothelial growth factor. *Endocr Rev*, 1997, 18, 4–25.

[34] McDonald, DM; Choyke, PL. Imaging of angiogenesis: from microscope to clinic. *Nat Med*, 2003, 9, 713–25.

[35] Achen, MG; Stacker, SA. The vascular endothelial growth factor family; proteins which guide the development of the vasculature. *Int J Exp Pathol*, 1998, 79, 255–65.

[36] Shibuya, M. Structure and function of VEGF/VEGF-receptor system involved in angiogenesis. *Cell Struct Funct*, 2001, 26, 25–35.

[37] Scotney, PD; MacKenzie, A; Maccarone, P; et al. Human vascular endothelial growth factor B: characterization of recombinant isoforms and generation of neutralizing monoclonal antibodies. Clin. Exp. Pharmacol. *Physiol*, 2002, 29 (11), 1024-1029.

[38] Carmeliet, P; Moons, L; Luttun, A; et al. Synergism between vascular endothelial growth factor and placental growth factor contributes to angiogenesis and plasma extravasation in pathological conditions. *Nat. Med.*, 2001, 7 (5), 575-583.

[39] Luttun, A; Tjwa, M; Moons, L; et al. Revascularization of ischemic tissues by PlGF treatment; and inhibition of tumor angiogenesis; arthritis and atherosclerosis by anti-Flt1. *Nat. Med.*, 2002, 8 (8), 831-840.

[40] Shibuya, M; Yamaguchi, S; Yamane, A; et al. Nucleotide sequence and expression of a novel human receptor-type tyrosine kinase gene (flt) closely related to the fms family *Oncogene*, 1990, 5 (4), 519-524.

[41] Takahashi, H; Shibuya, M. The vascular endothelial growth factor (VEGF)/VEGF receptor system and its role under physiological and pathological conditions. *Clin. Sci.*, 2005, 109(3), 227-241.

[42] Alitalo, K; Carmeliet, P. Molecular mechanisms of lymphangiogenesis in health and disease. *Cancer Cell*, 2002, 1 (3), 219-227.

[43] Veikkola, T; Jussila, L; Makinen, T; et al. Signalling via vascular endothelial growth factor receptor-3 is sufficient for lymphangiogenesis in transgenic mice. *EMBO J.*, 2001, 20 (6), 1223-1231.

[44] Fong, GH; Rossant, J; Gertsenstein, M; et al. Role of the Flt-1 receptor tyrosine kinase in regulating the assembly of vascular endothelium. *Nature* (London). 1995, 376 (6535), 66-70.

[45] Hiratsuka, S; Minowa, O; Kuno, J; et al. Flt-1 lacking the tyrosine kinase domain is sufficient fornormal development and angiogenesis in mice. *Proc. Natl. Acad. Sci. U.S.A.*, 1998, 95 (16), 9349-9354.

[46] Lin, EY; Li, JF; Gnatovskiy, L; et al. Macrophages regulate the angiogenic switch in a mouse model of breast cancer. *Cancer Res*, 2006, 66 (23):11238-11246.

[47] Murakami, M; Zheng, Y; Hirashima, M; et al. VEGFR1 tyrosine kinase signaling promotes lymphangiogenesis as well as angiogenesis indirectly via macrophage recruitment. Arterioscler. Thromb. *Vasc. Biol.*, 2008, 28, 658-664.

[48] Shalaby, F; Rossant, J; Yamaguchi, TP; et al. Failure of blood-island formation and vasculogenesis in Flk-1-deficient mice. *Nature* (London)., 1995, 376 (6535), 62-66.

[49] Petrova, TV; Makinen, T; Alitalo, K; et al. Signaling via vascular endothelial growth factor receptors. *Exp. Cell Res.*, 1999, 253 (1), 117-130.

[50] Tong, RT; Boucher, Y; Kozin, SV; et al. Vascular normalization by vascular endothelial growth factor receptor 2 blockadc induces a pressure gradient across the vasculature and improves drug penetration in tumors. *Cancer Res*, 2004, 64, 3731–6.

[51] Wildiers, H; Guetens, G; Boeck, GD; Verbeken, E; Landuyt, B; de Bruijn, EA; et al. Effect of antivascular endothelial growth factor treatment on the intratumoral uptake of CPT-11. *Br J Cancer*, 2003, 88, 1979–86.

[52] Jain, RK. Normalization of tumor vasculature: an emerging concept in antiangiogenic therapy. *Science*, 2005, 307, 58–62.

[53] Ferrara, N. Vascular endothelial growth factor as a target for anticancer therapy. *Oncologist*, 2004, 9, Suppl 1, 2^10.

[54] Kabbinavar, FF; Hambleton, J; Mass, RD; Hurwitz, HI; Bergsland, E; Sarkar, S. Combined analysis of efficacy: the addition of bevacizumab to fluorouracil/leucovorin improves survival for patientswith metastatic colorectal cancer. *J Clin Oncol.*, 2005, 23, 3706^12

[55] Giantonio, BJ; Catalano, PJ; Meropol, NJ; et al. Highdose bevacizumab improves survival when combined with FOLFOX4 in previously treated advanced colorectal cancer: results from the eastern cooperative oncology group (ECOG) study E3200. *J Clin Oncol*, 2005, 23, 1S.

[56] Hurwitz, H; Fehrenbacher, L; Novotny, W; et al. Bevacizumab plus irinotecan; fluorouracil; and leucovorin for metastatic colorectal cancer. *N. Engl. J. Med*, 2004, 350 (23), 2335–2342. First Phase III clinical trial of an antiangiogenic agent in metastatic colorectal cancer.

[57] Sandler, A; Gray, R; Perry, MC; et al. Paclitaxel–carboplatin alone or with bevacizumab for non-smallcell lung cancer. *N. Engl. J. Med*, 2006, 355(24), 2542–2550.

[58] Miller, K; Wang, M; Gralow, J; et al. Paclitaxel plus bevacizumab versus paclitaxel alone for metastatic breast cancer. *N. Engl. J. Med*, 2007, 357(26), 2666–2676. First Phase III clinical trial of bevacizumab in combination with chemotherapy as first-line therapy in metastatic breast cancer; which demonstrated a progression-free survival (PFS) benefit.

[59] Cloughesy, TF; Prados, MD; Wen, PY; et al. A Phase II; randomized; non-comparative clinical trial of the effect of bevacizumab (BV) alone or in combination with irinotecan (CPT) on 6-month progression free survival (PFS6) in recurrent; treatment-refractory glioblastoma (GBM). *J. Clin. Oncol*, 2008, 26 (Suppl) (Abstract 2010b).

[60] Jain, RK. Normalizing tumor vasculature with anti-angiogenic therapy. A new paradigm for combination therapy. *Nat Med.*, 2001, 7, 987–989.

[61] Willett, CG; et al. Direct evidence that the VEGF-specific antibody bevacizumab has antivascular effects in human rectal cancer. *Nat Med.*, 2004, 10, 145–147.

[62] Cobleigh, MA; Langmuir, VK; Sledge, GW; et al. A Phase I/II dose-escalation trial of bevacizumab in previously treated metastatic breast cancer. *Semin Oncol*, 2003, 30 (5 Suppl 16), 117–124.

[63] Midgley, R; Kerr, D: Bevacizumab-current status and future directions. *Ann Oncol*, 16, 999-1004, 2005.

[64] Dupont, J; Schwartz, L; Koutcher, D; Spriggs, DR; Gordon, MS; Mendelson, D; et al. Phase I and pharmacokinetic study of VEGF Trap

administered subcutaneously to patients with advanced solid malignancies. *Proc Am Soc Clin Oncol*, 2004, 23, 197 (#3009).

[65] Abrams, TJ; Lee, LB; Murray, LJ; Pryer, NK; Cherrington, JM. SU11248 inhibits KIT and platelet-derived growth factor receptor h in preclinical models of human small cell lung cancer. *Mol Cancer Ther*, 2003, 2, 471^8.

[66] O'Farrell, AM; Abrams, TJ; Yuen, HA; et al. SU11248 is a novel FLT3 tyrosine kinase inhibitor with potent activity in vitro and in vivo. *Blood*, 2003, 101, 3597^605.

[67] Faivre, S; Delbaldo, C; Vera, K; Robert, C; Lozahic, S; Lassau, N; et al. Safety; pharmacokinetic; and antitumor activity of SU11248, a novel oral multitarget tyrosin kinase inhibitor; in patients with cancer. *J Clin Oncol*, 2006, 24, 25–35.

[68] Starling, N; Vazquez, F; Cunningham, D; Chau, I; Ramos, FJ; Saunders, MP; et al. Phase I study to evaluate safety and efficacy of sunitinib in combination with FOLFIRI in treatment-naı¨ve metastatic colorectal cancer. *Proc Am Soc Clin Oncol*, 2008, 26, 15S (#3563).

[69] Arora, A; Scholar, EM. Role of tyrosine kinase inhibitors in cancer therapy. *J Pharmacol Exp Ther.*, 2005, 315, 971–979.

[70] Pawson, T. Regulation and targets of receptor tyrosine kinases. *Eur J Cancer.*, 2002, 38 (Suppl 5): S3–S10.

[71] Cheng, AL; et al. Efficacy and safety of sorafenib in patients in the Asia-Pacific region with advanced hepatocellular carcinoma: a phase III randomised; double-blind; placebo-controlled trial. *Lancet Oncol.*, 2009, 10, 25–34.

[72] Llovet, JM; et al. Sorafenib in advanced hepatocellular carcinoma. *N Engl J Med.*, 2008, 359, 378– 390.

[73] Morabito, A; De Maio, E; Di Maio, M; et al. Tyrosine kinase inhibitors of vascular endothelial growth factor receptors in clinical trials: current status and future directions. *Oncologist.*, 2006, 11 (7), 753-764.

[74] Gan, HK; Seruga, B; Knox, JJ. Sunitinib in solid tumors. Expert Opin. Investig. *Drugs.*, 2009, 18 (6), 821-834.

[75] Wilhelm, SM; Adnane, L; Newell, P; et al. Preclinical overview of sorafenib; a multikinase inhibitor that targets both Raf and VEGF and PDGF receptor tyrosine kinase signaling. Mol. *Cancer Ther.*, 2008, 7, 3129-3140.

[76] Clark, JW; Eder, JP; Ryan, D; et al. Safety and pharmacokinetics of the dual action raf kinase and vascular endothelial growth factor receptor

inhibitor; BAY 43-9006, in patients with advanced; refractory solid tumors. *Clin Cancer Res*, 2005, 11, 5472–80.

[77] Minami, H; Kawada, K; Ebi, H; et al. Phase I and pharmacokinetic study of sorafenib; an oral multikinase inhibitor; in Japanese patients with advanced refractory solid tumors. *Cancer Sci*, 2008, 99, 1492–8.

[78] Hutson, TE; Davis, ID; Machiels, JP; et al. Efficacy and Safety of Pazopanib in Patients With Metastatic Renal Cell Carcinoma. *J Clin Oncol.*, 2010, 28 (3), 475–480.

[79] Sleijfer, S; Ray-Coquard, I; Papai, Z; et al. Pazopanib; a multikinase angiogenesis inhibitor; in patients with relapsed or refractory advanced soft tissue sarcoma: a phase II study from the European organisation for research and treatment of cancer-soft tissue and bone sarcoma group (EORTC study 62043). *J Clin Oncol.*, 2009, 27 (19), 3126–3132.

[80] Sternberg, CN; Szczylik, C; Lee, E; et al. A randomized; double-blind phase III study of pazopanib in treatment-naive and cytokine-pretreated patients with advanced renal cell carcinoma (RCC). *J Clin Oncol.*, 2009, 27, 15s(Suppl):abstr 5021.

[81] Seger, R; Krebs, EG. The MAPK signaling cascade. *FASEB J.* 1995, 9(9): 726–735. Dhillon AS; Hagan S; Rath O; Kolch W. MAP kinase signaling pathways in cancer. *Oncogene.*, 2007, 26 (22), 3279–3290.

[82] Poulikakos, PI; Zhang, C; Bollag, G; Shokat, KM; Rosen, N. RAF inhibitors transactivate RAF dimers and ERK signalling in cells with wild-type BRAF. *Nature.*, 2010, 464, 427–430.

[83] Bhatt, KV; Spofford, LS; Aram, G; et al. Adhesion control of cyclin D1 and p27Kip1 levels is deregulated in melanoma cells through BRAF-MEK-ERK signaling. *Oncogene. May*, 12, 2005, 24 (21), 3459–71.

[84] Paik, PK; Arcila, ME; Fara, M; et al. Clinical characteristics of patients with lung adenocarcinomas harboring BRAF mutations. *J Clin Oncol.*, 2011, 29, 2046–2051.

[85] Santarpia, L; Qi, Y; Stemke-Hale, K; et al. Mutation profiling identifies numerous rare drug targets and distinct mutation patterns in different clinical subtypes of breast cancers. *Breast Cancer Res Treat.*, 2012, 134, 333–343.

[86] Singer, G; Kurman, RJ; Chang, HW; et al. Diverse tumorigenic pathways in ovarian serous carcinoma. *Am J Pathol.*, 2002, 160, 1223–1228.

[87] Singer, G; Oldt, R; 3rd; Cohen, Y; et al. Mutations in BRAF and KRAS characterize the development of low-grade ovarian serous carcinoma. *J Natl Cancer Inst.*, 2003, 95, 484–486.

[88] Sieben, NL; Macropoulos, P; Roemen, GM; et al. In ovarian neoplasms; BRAF; but not KRAS; mutations are restricted to low-grade serous tumours. *J Pathol.*, 2004, 202, 336–340.

[89] Kimura, ET; Nikiforova, MN; Zhu, Z; et al. High prevalence of BRAF mutations in thyroid cancer: genetic evidence for constitutive activation of the RET/PTC-RAS-BRAF signaling pathway in papillary thyroid carcinoma. *Cancer Res.*, 2003, 63, 1454–1457. Drug; Healthcare and Patient Safety 2014, 6

[90] Lupi, C; Giannini, R; Ugolini, C; et al. Association of BRAF V600E mutation with poor clinicopathological outcomes in 500 consecutive cases of papillary thyroid carcinoma. *J Clin Endocrinol Metab.*, 2007, 92, 4085–4090.

[91] Kalady, MF; Dejulius, KL; Sanchez, JA; et al. BRAF mutations in colorectal cancer are associated with distinct clinical characteristics and worse prognosis. *Dis Colon Rectum.*, 2012, 55 (2):128–133.

[92] Frasca, F; Nucera, C; Pellegriti, G; et al. BRAF (V600E) mutation and the biology of papillary thyroid cancer. *Endocr Relat Cancer.*, 2008, 15 (2), 191–205.

[93] Tiacci, E; Trifonov, V; Schiavoni, G; et al. BRAFmutations in hairy-cell leukemia. *N Engl J Med*, 2011, 364, 2305–15.

[94] Brose, MS; Volpe, P; Feldman, M; et al. BRAF and RAS mutations in human lung cancer and melanoma. *Cancer Res.*, 2002, 62 (23), 6997–7000.

[95] Long, GV; Menzies, AM; Nagrial, AM; et al. Prognostic and clinicopathologic associations of oncogenic BRAF in metastatic melanoma. *J Clin Oncol.*, 2011, 29 (10), 1239-1246.

[96] Shinozaki, M; Fujimoto, A; Morton, DL; et al. Incidence of BRAF oncogene mutation and clinical relevance for primary cutaneous melanomas. *Clin Cancer Res.*, 2004, 10, 1753–1757.

[97] Maldonado, JL; Fridlyand, J; Patel, H; et al. Determinants of BRAF mutations in primary melanomas. *J Natl Cancer Inst.*, 2003, 95, 1878–1890.

[98] Wan, PT; Garnett, MJ; Roe, SM; et al. Mechanism of activation of the RAF-ERK signaling pathway by oncogenic mutations of B-RAF. *Cell.*, 2004, 116 (6), 855–867.

[99] Moreau, S; Saiag, P; Aegerter, P; et al. Prognostic value of BRAF (V600) mutations in m9lanoma patients after resection of metastatic lymph nodes. *Ann Surg Oncol. Epub July*, 7, 2012.

[100] Kumar, R; Angelini, S; Czene, K; et al. BRAF mutations in metastatic melanoma: a possible association with clinical outcome. *Clin Cancer Res*, 2003, 9, 3362–8.

[101] Tsai, J; Lee, JT; Wang, W; et al. Discovery of a selective inhibitor of oncogenic B-Raf kinase with potent antimelanoma activity. *Proc Natl Acad Sci U S A.*, 2008, 105 (8), 3041–3046.

[102] Tronnier, M; Mitteldorf, C. Treating advanced melanoma: current insights and opportunities. *Cancer Management and Research*, 2014, 6 349–356

[103] Wellbrock, C; Ogilvie, L; Hedley, D; et al. V599EBRAF is an oncogene in melanocytes. *Cancer Res*, 2004, 64 (7), 2338–42.

[104] Hingorani, SR; Jacobetz, MA; Robertson, GP; et al. Suppression of BRAF(V599E) in human melanoma abrogates transformation. *Cancer Research.*, 2003, 63 (17), 5198–202.

[105] Zhang, J; Yang, PL; Gray, NS. Targeting cancer with small molecule kinase inhibitors. *Nat Rev Cancer.*, 2009, 9 (1), 28–39.

[106] Liu, Y; Gray. Rational design of inhibitors that bind to inactive kinase conformations. *Nat Chem Biol.*, 2006, 2, 358–364.

[107] Wilhelm, SM; Carter, C; Tang, L; et al. BAY 43-9006 exhibits broad spectrum oral antitumor activity and targets the RAF/MEK/ERK pathway and receptor tyrosine kinases involved in tumor progression and angiogenesis. *Cancer Res*, 2004, 64 (19): 7099–109.

[108] Wilhelm, SM; Adnane, L; Newell, P; et al. Preclinical overview of sorafenib; a multikinase inhibitor that targets both Raf and VEGF and PDGF receptor tyrosine kinase signaling. *Mol Cancer Ther*, 2008, 7, 3129–40.

[109] Flaherty, KT; Redlinger, M; Schuchter, LM; et al. Phase I/II; pharmacokinetic and pharmacodynamic trial of BAY 43-9006 alone in patients with metastatic melanoma. *J Clin Oncol.*, 2005, 23(16 Suppl): Abstract 3037.

[110] Min, CJ; Liebes, LF; Escalon, J; et al. Phase II trial of sorafenib in metastatic melanoma including detection of BRAF with mutant specific-PCR and altered proliferation pathways-final outcome analysis. *J Clin Oncol*, 26, 2008 (suppl; abstr 9072).

[111] Flaherty, KT; Schiller, J; Schuchter, LM; et al. A phase I trial of the oral; multikinase inhibitor sorafenib in combination with carboplatin and paclitaxel. *Clin Cancer Res*. 2008, 14 (15):4836–4842. Ott PA; Hamilton A; Min C; et al. A phase II trial of sorafenib in metastatic melanoma with tissue correlates. *PLoS One.*, 2010, 5 (12), e1558.

[112] Amaravadi, RK; Schuchter, LM; McDermott, DF; et al. Phase II trial of temozolomide and sorafenib in advanced melanoma patients with or without brain metastases. *Clin Cancer Res*, 2009, 15, 7711–8.
[113] Flaherty, KT; Puzanov, I; Kim, KB; et al. Chapman PB. Inhibition of mutated; activated BRAF in metastatic melanoma. *N Engl J Med*, 2010, 363, 809–19.
[114] Eisen, T; Ahmad, T; Flaherty, KT; et al. Sorafenib in advanced melanoma: a Phase II randomised discontinuation trial analysis. *Br J Cancer. Sep*, 4, 2006 95 (5), 581–6.
[115] Hauschild, A; Agarwala, SS; Trefzer, U; et al. Results of a phase III; randomized; placebo-controlled study of sorafenib in combination with carboplatin and paclitaxel as second-line treatment in patients with unresectable stage III or stage IV melanoma. *J Clin Oncol.*, 2009, 27, 2823.30.
[116] Bollag, G; Hirth, P; Tsai, J; et al. Clinical efficacy of a RAF inhibitor needs broad target blockade in BRAF-mutant melanoma. *Nature.*, 2010, 467(7315), 596–599.
[117] Flaherty, KT; Puzanov, I; Sosman, J; et al. Phase I study of PLX4032, proof of concept for V600E BRAF mutation as a therapeutic target in human cancer. *J Clin Oncol*, 2009, 27, 15S.
[118] Eggermont, AMM. Advances in systemic treatment of melanoma. Annals of Oncology 21 (Supplement 7): vii339–vii344, 2010.
[119] Sosman, JA; Kim, KB; Schuchter, L; et al. Survival in BRAF V600-mutant advanced melanoma treated with vemurafenib. *N Engl J Med.* 2012, 366(8), 707–714.
[120] Slipicevic, A; Herlyn, M. Narrowing the knowledge gaps for melanoma. *Ups J Med Sci.*, 2012, 117, 237-43
[121] Tsai, KY; Nowroozi, S; Kim, KB. Drug safety evaluation of vemurafenib in the treatment of melanoma. Expert Opin Drug Saf. 2013, 12(5):767-75. Jang S; and Atkins MB. Treatment of BRAF-Mutant Melanoma: The Role of Vemurafenib and Other Therapies. *Clin Pharmacol Ther.*, 2014, 95 (1), 24-31.
[122] Foletto, MC; Haas, SE. Cutaneous melanoma: new advances in treatment. *An Bras Dermatol.*, 2014, 89 (2), 301-10.
[123] Dummer, R; Goldinger, SM; Turtschi, CP; et al. Vemurafenib in patients with BRAF(V600) mutation-positive melanoma with symptomatic brain metastases: final results of an open-label pilot study. *Eur J Cancer.*, 2014 Feb, 50 (3), 611-21.

[124] Sosman, JA; Kim, KB; Schuchter, L; et al. Survival in BRAF V600–Mutant Advanced Melanoma Treated with Vemurafenib. *N Engl J Med.*, 2012, 366 (8), 707–714.

[125] Chapman, PB; Hauschild, A; Robert, C; et al. Improved survival with vemurafenib in melanoma with BRAF V600E mutation. *N Engl J Med.*, 2011, 364(26), 2507-16.

[126] McArthur, GA; Chapman, PB; Robert, C; et al. Safety and efficacy of vemurafenib in BRAF (V600E) and BRAF (V600K) mutation-positive melanoma (BRIM-3): extended follow-up of a phase 3, randomised; open-label study. *Lancet Oncol.*, 2014, 15, 323–332.

[127] Kudchadkar, RR; Gonzalez, R; Lewis, K. New Targeted Therapies in Melanoma. *Cancer Control.*, 2013, 20(4), 282-8.

[128] Mcgettigan, S. Dabrafenib: A New Therapy for Use in BRAF-Mutated Metastatic Melanoma *J Adv Pract Oncol*, 2014, 5, 211–215.

[129] Argenziano, G; Lallas, A; Longo, C; et al. Dormant melanomas or changing nevi? *J Invest Dermatol.*, 2014, 134(5), 1196–1198.

[130] Laquerre, S; Arnone, M; Moss, K; et al. A selective Raf kinase inhibitor induces cell death and tumor regression of human cancer cell lines encoding B-RafV600E mutation. *Mol Cancer Ther.*, 2009, 12 Suppl 1, Abstr B88.

[131] Wagle, N; Emery, C; Berger, MF; et al. Dissecting therapeutic resistance to RAF inhibition in melanoma by tumor genomic profiling. *J Clin Oncol.*, 2011, 29, 3085–3096.

[132] Shi, H; Moriceau, G; Kong, X; et al. Melanoma whole-exome sequencing identifies (V600E)B-RAF amplification-mediated acquired B-RAF inhibitor resistance. *Nat Commun.*, 2012, 3, 724.

[133] Straussman, R; Morikawa, T; Shee, K; et al. Tumour micro-environment elicits innate resistance to RAF inhibitors through HGF secretion. *Nature.*, 2012, 487, 500–504.

[134] McArthur, GA; Ribas, A; Chapman, PB; et al. Molecular analyses from a phase I trial of vemurafenib to study mechanism of action and resistance in repeated biopsies from BRAF mutation—positive metastatic melanoma patients. *J Clin Oncol*, 29, 2011 (suppl; abstr 8502).

[135] Poulikakos, PI; Persaud, Y; Janakiraman, M; et al. RAF inhibitor resistance is mediated by dimerization of aberrantly spliced BRAF(V600E). *Nature*, 2011, 480, 387–90.

[136] Montagut, C; Sharma, SV; Shioda, T; et al. Elevated CRAF as a potential mechanism of acquired resistance to BRAF inhibition in melanoma. *Cancer Res*, 2008, 68, 4853–61.

[137] Kaplan, FM; Shao, Y; Mayberry, MM; et al. Hyperactivation of MEKERK1/2 signaling and resistance to apoptosis induced by the oncogenic B-RAF inhibitor; PLX4720, in mutant N-RAS melanoma cells. *Oncogene*, 2011, 30, 366–71.

[138] Hatzivassiliou, G; Song, K; Yen, I; et al. RAF inhibitors prime wild-type RAF to activate the MAPK pathway and enhance growth. *Nature.*, 2010, 464, 431–435.

[139] Heidorn, SJ; Milagre, C; Whittaker, S; et al. Kinase-dead BRAF and oncogenic RAS cooperate to drive tumor progression through *CRAF. Cell.*, 2010, 140, 209–221.

[140] Hahn, WC; Garraway, LA. COT drives resistance to RAF inhibition through MAP kinase pathway reactivation. *Nature*, 2010, 468, 968–72.

[141] Holderfield, M; Merritt, H; Chan, J; et al. RAF inhibitors activate the MAPK pathway by relieving inhibitory autophosphorylation. *Cancer Cell.*, 2013, 23, 594–602.

[142] Paraiso, KH; Fedorenko, IV; Cantini, LP; et al. Recovery of phospho-ERK activity allows melanoma cells to escape from BRAF inhibitor therapy. *Br J Cancer*, 2010, 102, 1724–30.

[143] Smalley, KS; Lioni, M; Palma, MD; et al. Increased cyclin D1 expression can mediate BRAF inhibitor resistance in BRAF V600E-mutated melanomas. *Mol Cancer Ther.*, 2008, 7 (9), 2876–83.

[144] Paraiso, KH; Xiang, Y; Rebecca, VW; et al. PTEN loss confers BRAF inhibitor resistance to melanoma cells through the suppression of BIM expression. *Cancer Res.*, 2011, 71 (7), 2750–60.

[145] Xing, F; Persaud, Y; Pratilas, CA; et al. Concurrent loss of the PTEN and RB1 tumor suppressors attenuates RAF dependence in melanomas harboring (V600E)BRAF. *Oncogene.*, 2012, 31 (4), 446-57.

[146] Sawyers, C. Targeted cancer therapy. *Nature*. Nov, 18, 2004, 432 (7015), 294–7.

[147] Shi, H; Hong, A; Kong, X; et al. A novel AKT1 mutant amplifies an adaptive melanoma response to BRAF inhibition. *Cancer Discov.*, 2014, 4, 69-79.

[148] Nazarian, R; Shi, H; Wang, Q; et al. Melanomas acquire resistance to B-RAF (V600E) inhibition by RTK or N-RAS upregulation. *Nature.*, 2010, 468 (7326), 973–977.

[149] Flaherty, KT; Infante, JR; Daud, A; et al. Combined BRAF and MEK inhibition in melanoma with BRAF V600 mutations. *N Engl J Med.*, 2012, 367 (18), 1694-1703.

In: New Skin Toxicities …
Editors: Giulia Ganzetti et al.
ISBN: 978-1-63482-224-4

Chapter 2

Skin Toxicities from EGFR Inhibitors

G. Ganzetti*, MD and A. Offidani, MD, Professor
Dermatology Unit, Department of Clinical and Molecular Sciences, Polytechnic Marche University, Italy

Abstract

The last few years have signed the introduction of EGFR inhibitors in the treatment of several types of cancers, as non-small cell lung cancer and head neck malignancies. This class of drugs comprises monoclonal antibodies (cetuximab, panitumumab) and tyrosine kinase inhibitors (erlotinib and gefitinib).

Although generally well tolerated, these targeted drugs are related to muco-cutaneous adverse reactions in a significant number of treated patients. Papulo-pustular rash, also known as acneiform rash, is the most frequent adverse event which considerably influences patient's quality of life. This skin effect appears to be directly linked to the inhibition of EGFR action, despite the exact pathophysiology remains elusive.

Actually, no standardized guidelines are available for the management of EGFR-inhibitors' skin toxicities. Although the permanent drug discontinuation is rare, management of EGFR inhibitors' related

* Correspondence to: giulia.ganzetti@alice.it.

toxicities needs a multidisciplinary approach and represents a great challenge for dermatologists who face these clinical entities.

EGFR inhibitors represent a new important therapeutic strategy in cancer management. Also known as EGFR targeted therapy, they are able to selectively interfere on specific molecular targets reducing systemic toxicity and ensuring an improved safety profile [1].

Their use, in monotherapy or in combination with chemo/radio/hormone therapy, has greatly improved the treatment of many cancers and the patient's survival and quality of life [2].

Despite the incidence of systemic adverse events appears reduced, the wider use of EGFR-Is in clinical practice and the tight follow-up of the patients have led to the identification of EGFR-Is- mediated specific side effects [3].

These adverse effects may be associated with the worsen of patients' quality of life and their severity can lead to dose-reduction or to drug discontinuation, which could be permanent in 8-17% of cases [1].

The skin and the skin appendages are closely dependent to EGFR-mediated pathway [1].

Therefore, muco-cutaneous skin toxicities related to EGFR-inhibitors are principally characterized by papulo-pustular rash, cutaneous xerosis, nail dystrophy, itching, abnormal hair growth, hyperpigmentation, trichomegalia, telangiectasia and mucositis [4].

Therefore an appropriate multidisciplinary diagnostic-therapeutic approach of EGFR-Is' skin toxicities appears necessary to reach a consensus on patient's management [5].

EGFR and the Skin

EGFR is constitutively expressed in epidermal keratinocytes, in the outer sheath of the hair follicles, in sebocytes, in dendritic cells and in connective tissue cells.

EGFR participates to the skin physiology, in particular it:

- stimulates keratinocytes' proliferation and differentiation,
- accelerates wound healing,
- promotes the keratinocytes' migration through the expression of integrin α2,

- stimulates the turnover of phosphatidyl-inositol and diacylglycerol
- activates phospholipase A2 and prostaglandin E1,
- promotes vasoconstriction [6].

Before EGFR-Is treatment, the epidermal basal layer shows the expression of phosphorylated EGFR, the MAPK and the Ki67, a marker of cell proliferation; the keratin 1 (KRT1), the p27 (cyclin-dependent-kinase inhibitor, cell cycle inhibitory protein) and STAT3 (signal transducer and activator of transcription 3) are evidenced in the overlying layers.

After treatment with EGFR-Is, the loss of phosphorylated EGFR and the reduction of MAPK expression are identified. These two aspects are linked to the cell growth arrest and to an early cell differentiation, as demonstrated by the up-regulation of p27kip1, KRT1 and STAT3 and by the down-regulation of MAPK and Ki67 [7].

The premature keratinocyte differentiation is associated to the epidermal thinning and to reduced skin barrier function; in some cases, parakeratosis is evident [7-9].

Subsequently, the recruitment of inflammatory cells and the production of pro-inflammatory cytokines promote skin inflammation; furthermore, an increase in the keratinocytes' apoptosis, in tissue damage and in blood vessels' dilation occur. In particular, keratinocytes' apoptosis is increased by five times between 4-12th day of treatment; this period is directly related with the rash onset in treated patients [7-10].

Skin Rash (Figures 4, 5, 6)

The skin rash is the most frequent adverse event characterized by a papulo-pustular acneiform-like eruption, which occurs from 50 to 100% of patients treated with EGFR inhibitors [11].

Papulo-pustular rash tend to be more severe and widespread with monoclonal antibodies compared to small-molecule tyrosine kinase inhibitors and cetuximab is the most frequently EGFR-Is involved [12].

The frequency and the extent of the rash seem to be strictly related to the dose and the duration of the anti-neoplastic treatment [13].

Literature data have emphasized a strong correlation between the presence and severity of the eruption and the patients' survival; in fact, "*dose to rash*" studies have underlined that patients developing the skin rash during EGFR-Is appear to be most responsive to treatment. Therefore, acneiform rash may be considered a marker of the efficacy of the anti-neoplastic target therapy, as well as a predictor of disease-free survival [13, 14].

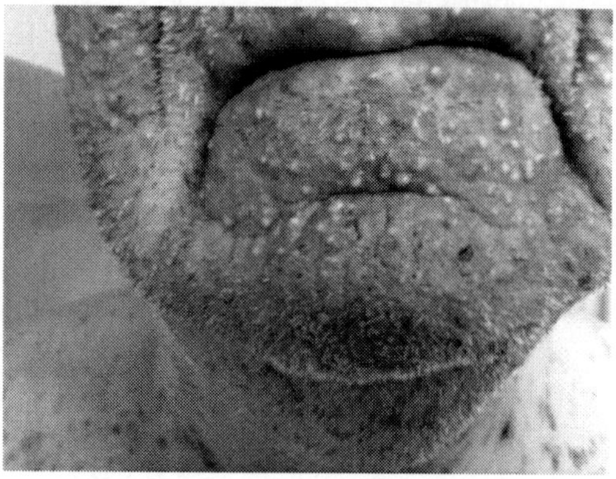

Figure 4.

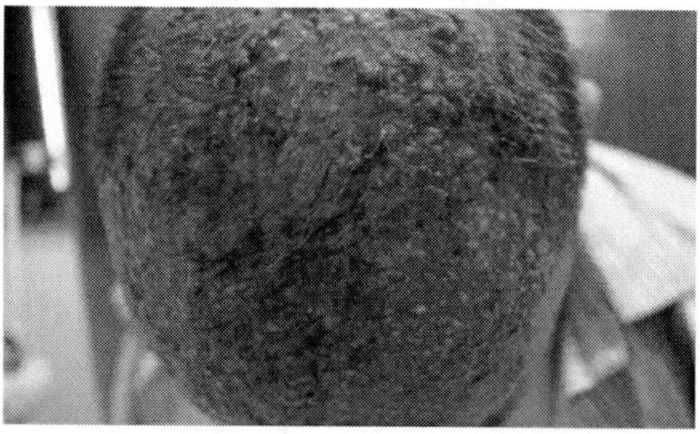

Figure 5.

Figure 6.

Although the lesions usually occur 1-2 weeks after the first dose of treatment, in some cases the onset may be within 2 days or later within 6 weeks. The rash can spontaneously heal during the treatment or 4-8 weeks after the drug discontinuation with dry hyperpigmented outcomes; however, a flare-up may occur after each infusion and the severity of the skin rash may decrease with long-term treatment. In severe cases, dose reduction or drug discontinuation or withdrawal should be considered [5, 11, 13].

Clinically, the lesions are represented by erythematous papules evolving into follicular pustular lesions or merging into plaques. Cutaneous lesions are similar to acne vulgaris, although some elements can help the clinicians to differ these two dermatological diseases. In fact, the EGFR-Is skin rash does not show blackheads, the pustular lesions are sterile and the scalp can be involved; moreover, the patient complains discomfort, itching, burning sensation and sometimes pain [15].

Skin lesions typically occur on seborrheic areas (face, scalp, trunk) and/or sun-exposed areas, sparing palms and soles; upper and lower limbs, abdomen and buttocks are rarely involved. The face is the most frequently affected area except for the skin reaction due to Lapatinib, which seems to prefer the trunk [16, 17].

Moreover, skin rash could be similar to rosacea, to seborrhoeic dermatitis or to cellulitis [15].

No correlations have been observed between the occurrence and severity of the skin rash and the patient's susceptibility for acne, seborrheic dermatitis and rosacea [18].

The development of the rash follows three principal steps:

- the first phase consists in erythema and edema accompanied to sensory disturbances, as itching and burning sensation
- the second phase is characterized by the onset of the papulo-pustular eruption
- the third phase is characterized by clinical outcomes as telangiectasia and hyperpigmentation [19].

As stated before, the papulo-pustular lesions are sterile; however, Staphylococcus Aureus and, rarely, viral or fungal infection can be identified secondary to scratching [18].

Similarly, the detection of Propionibacterium acnes or Malassezia furfur has been considered a pre-existent and independent event from the skin rash [18].

Histopathological evaluation of the lesions shows a non-specific suppurated aseptic folliculitis. In the earliest stages of EGFR-Is treatment, the inflammatory infiltrate is composed primarily of T cells, subsequently replaced by a dermal “bulky” neutrophilic infiltrate [20].

The horny layer appears thinned with the loss of the classic "basket” pattern; furthermore, the follicles are dilated and frequently filled by an excess of keratinocytes, as a consequence of the apoptosis inhibition and of the alteration of cells migration [20].

The inflammatory infiltrate leads to the tissue damage with acantholysis, degeneration of the keratinocytes of the epidermal basal layer and the destruction of the basal membrane [11].

Immunohistochemical studies and in situ hybridization have detected an increased expression of p27kip1 in the lesional skin. This molecule is a negative regulator of the cell cycle and, in physiological condition, it is only occasionally expressed by keratinocytes of the epidermal basal layer. Patients treated with EGFR-Is show a p27kip1 over-expression in all epidermal layers and a dermal-epidermal reduced expression of Ki67 and of Akt [11, 13, 21].

Nail Toxicity (Figures 7, 8)

The nail toxicity is less common than the skin rash and it has been observed in about 10-20% of treated patients, especially during the treatment with Cetuximab and Gefitinib [23].

Nail toxicity develops after a period ranging from 4-8 weeks to 6 months from the first dose.

The pathogenesis of paronychia has not been completely elucidated: it has been proposed that EGFR-Is may directly inhibit keratinocytes in the nail matrix. Moreover, it seems to be linked to skin fragility, which would facilitate the toenails’ ingrown and the inflammation of periungual tissue. Despite cultural exams have detected the Staphylococcus Aureus infection, it seems not achieve a significant impact in the pathogenesis of nail toxicity [22].

Recently, it has also been hypothesized that the growth of granulation tissue may be related to the lesional over-expression of angiogenetic factors, as VEGF (Vascular Endothelial Growth Factor). This aspect is still debated because it is known that EGFR-Is inhibit the VEGF expression and angiogenesis [22].

Paronychia can involve many fingers and toes and the big toe, in particular, is the most frequently affected [5].

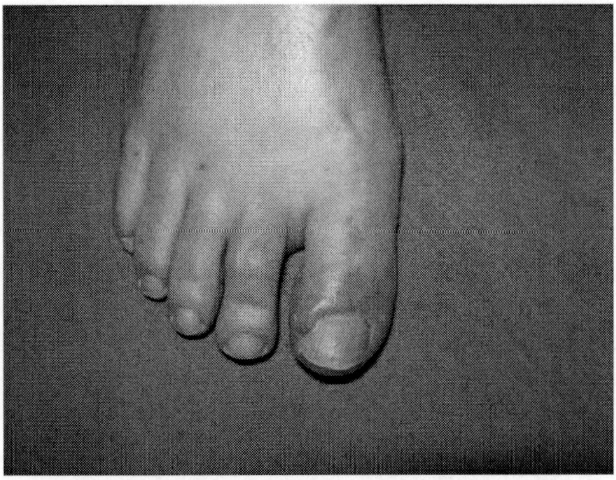

Figure 7.

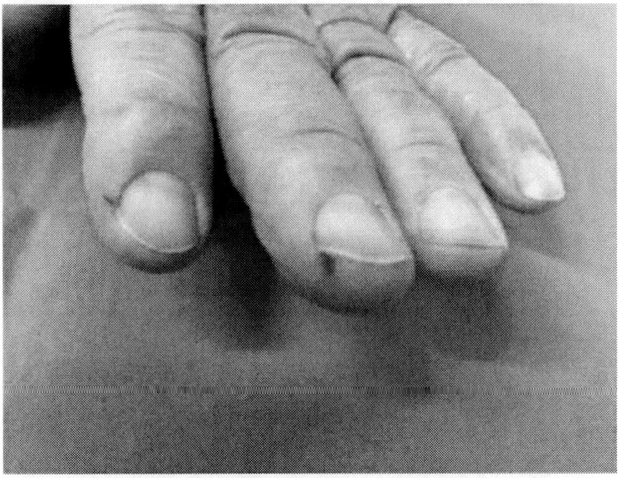

Figure 8.

Periungual tissue appears swollen, erythematous and painful, especially if nails' impaired growth occur with significant functional disability and obvious repercussions on patients' quality of life.

Abscesses and pyogenic granuloma-like lesions can complicate the clinical manifestation with possible associated infection due to Staphylococcus Aureus, Pseudomonas Aeruginosa and Candida albicans. The nail's growth is slower and nails appear extremely fragile with frequent onycholysis [5].

Most of patients developing nail toxicity show skin rash.

Histopathological evaluation of paronychia evidences wide dermal inflammation with an inflammatory infiltrate mainly consisting of plasma cells, lymphocytes and neutrophils, with prominent capillaries and stromal edema [5, 22, 24, 25].

Xerosis (Figures 8, 9, 10)

Xerosis affects more than 35% of patients during treatment with EGFR inhibitors; few reports have underlined that xerosis could be the leading skin adverse event with a prevalence of approximately 50% to 100% [26, 27].

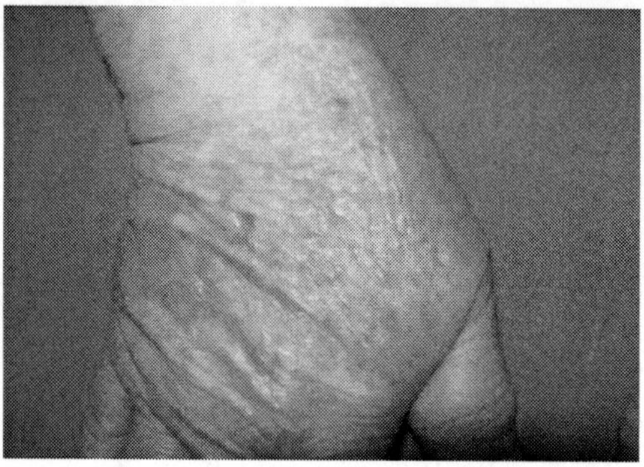

Figure 9.

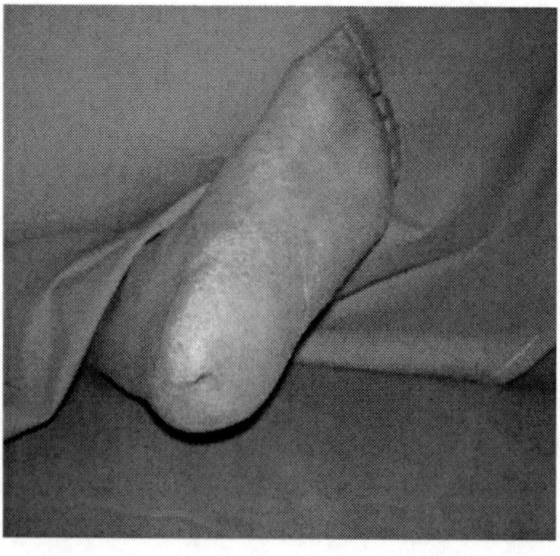

Figure 10.

Older age, atopy and previous treatment with cytotoxic agents represent concomitant risk factors for the development of xerosis during targeted therapy. The same areas previously affected by the acneiform eruption are involved: skin is dry, scaly and itchy and itching can vary from moderate to severe and tends to persist even after the drug discontinuation [15].

Xerosis may gradually evolve into a real asteatotic eczema and it could be complicated by secondary bacterial (Staphylococcus Aureus) or more rarely viral (Herpes virus) infections [18].

Sometimes a dry pulpitis with fingertips' painful fissures can be detected [18].

Mucous membranes may be invoved, in particular the vagina and perineum, with discomfort during urination [18].

The pathogenesis of xerosis appears to be linked to the skin barrier modifications due to EGFR-Is therapy. Numerous studies have shown that EGFR Knock-out mice tend to develop dry skin, with decreased loricrin production in epidermal granulosum layer [28].

Loricrin plays a pivotal role in maintaining epidermal barrier function counteracting the trans-epidermal water loss [28].

Hyperpigmentation (Figure 11)

Hyperpigmentation is manly observed in patients treated with Gefitinib [23].

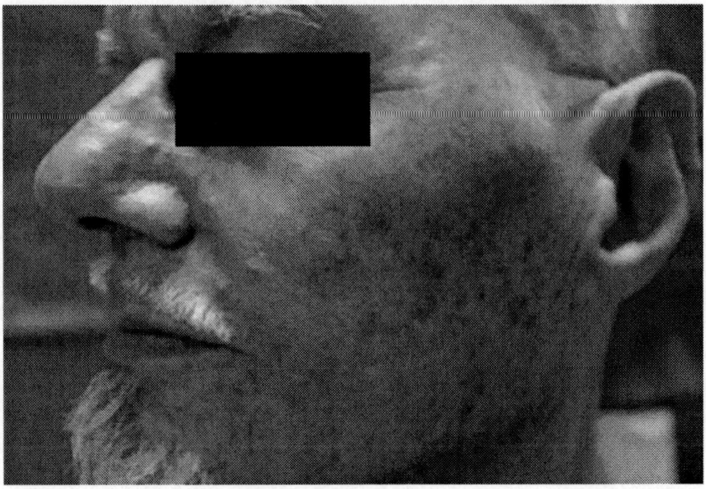

Figure 11.

It generally presents as hyperpigmented outcome secondary to acneiform eruption or to eczema, thus it involves the face, the trunk, the lower limbs, even several months after treatment with EGFR inhibitors [26].

Sun exposure worsen hyperpigmented outcomes [23, 26].

Histological examination shows a pigment increase in the basal keratinocytes with melanin engulfed by macrophages of the superficial dermis. The pathogenesis of hyperpigmentation is probably due to a sort of transfer of a larger melanin amount in basal keratinocytes and dermal macrophages as secondary post-inflammatory effect [23].

Abnormalities of Hair Growth (Figure 12)

Hair growth alterations are rarely observed in 5-6% of patients treated with EGFR inhibitors.

It is known that EGFR is localized in the outer sheath of the hair follicles, interfering with hair growth cycle, hair orientation and elongation. It is known that the hair cycle is principally divided into three phases, anagen, catagen and telogen, which respectively correspond to the phase of growth, regression and rest. The EGFR is able to stimulate and modulate the transition from the anagen phase to the catagen phase [5, 16, 26, 29].

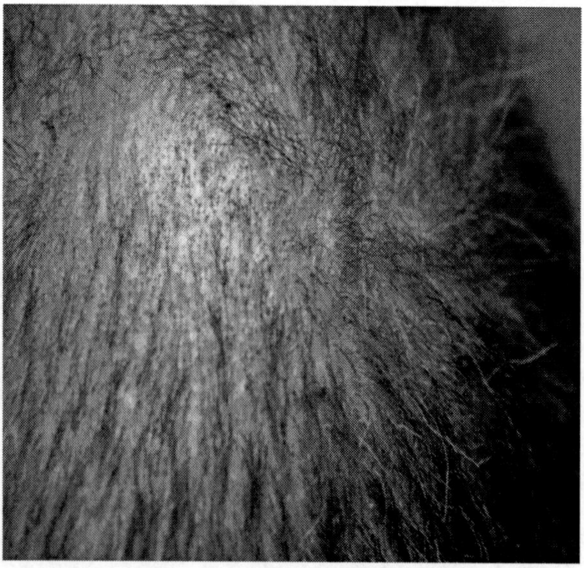

Figure 12.

Clinical manifestations vary according to the anatomical area. In fact, face is most commonly affected by trichomegaly and hypertrichosis, due to an excessive and abnormal hair growth, whereas the extremities and the scalp present alopecia, which is the expression of an anagen phase alteration [30].

Trichomegaly usually develops 2-5 months after initiating EGFR-Is and generally resolves within 1 month after drug withdrawal [30].

This uncommon adverse event is mainly described in patients affected by colorectal carcinoma or lung carcinoma and treated with Cetuximab or Erlotinib [31].

It consists on hair length increase, stiffness and pigmentation in malar region and lips; the eyelashes appear extremely thin, curly and aberrant and it may lead to corneal irritation and ulceration. In some cases, it is accompanied by poliosis which consists in melanin loss [31].

As regards the scalp, hair abnormalities consist of hair growth reduction leading to fragile and curly hairs with both scarring and non-scarring inflammatory alopecia [32, 33].

Hair loss occur months or years after the first dose of EGFR-Is therapy, especially in patients treated with combination therapy of EGFR-Is and Irinotecan [32, 33].

Non-scarring alopecia has been recorded in patients treated with Gefitinib and it is linked to both hair growth arrest and to the intense inflammatory reaction [5, 23, 32, 33]. Although the pathogenetic mechanism has not been completely clarified, it seems to be due to the increased terminal differentiation due to EGFR inhibition [34].

Teleangiectasia

Teleangiectasias can occur during the early stages of the skin rash or during the skin rash flare-up in the face, the ear, the trunk, the chest, the lumbar region [9, 23]. After their gradual improvement, teleangiectasias can leave hyperpigmented outcomes [9, 23].

The onset of telangiectasia seems to be linked to an abnormal production of angiogenetic factors such as VEGF (Vascular Endothelial Growth Factor) [35].

Photosensitivity

EGFR inhibitors have photosensitizing properties and some patients may develop diffuse erythema, papules and pustules in sun-exposed areas; however, severe bullous lesions are rare [36].

The photosensitivity is related to the amplification of UV-mediated damage. It is known that ultraviolet radiations are responsible for keratinocytes' damage through the formation of thymine dimers and the production of reactive oxygen species; moreover, they also activate the EGFR-mediated signal leading to an increased epidermal proliferation [37].

Mucositis

Mucositis is a rare adverse event occurring when EGFR-Is are used in combination with traditional chemotherapy or radiation therapy.

Oral mucosa is involved with aphtoid-like lesions that are often complicated by fungal infections (Candida albicans).

Moreover, erosions, angular cheilitis can be identified as well as geographic tongue, which is characterized by erythematous patches with a raised white-yellow serpiginous border.

Patients can complain dysgeusia and xerostomia.

Nasal mucosa can be involved with epistaxis, whereas vulvo-vaginitis and balanitis can be diagnosed in genital mucosae [35, 38, 39].

Therapeutic Management of Skin Toxicities

Therapeutic management of EGFR-Is related skin toxicities include both general prophylactic measures and specific treatments targeting each clinical manifestation [41].

Each patient, who is candidate to EGFR inhibitors, should undergo to a careful dermatological clinical examination in order to highlight a previous or a current history of xerosis, acne vulgaris or atopic dermatitis.

Furthermore, in order to reduce the risk of skin toxicity, some general measures are suggested as the use of delicate cleansing products avoiding hygiene products containing alcohol, such as lotions or perfumes that can cause irritation and/or exacerbate the xerosis. Moreover, synthetic clothing and tight shoes should be avoided preferring natural fibers and comfortable shoes.

To prevent xerosis and trans-epidermal water loss, the use of emollients appears to be an important element; moreover, the bath should be of short duration and with warm water to reduce the risk of dehydration.

Finally, sun exposure should be strictly controlled and the use of highly protective sunscreen (Sun Protection Factor SPF greater than 30) is mandatory; physical filters containing zinc oxide or titanium dioxide are preferred to chemical ones in order to reduce skin irritation.

All these measures are useful both to decrease the risk of onset and the flare-up of the papular-pustular rash and to limit hyperpigmented outcomes.

Finally, manicures and pedicures should be avoided to the prevent superinfections and ingrown nails [40, 42, 43].

Specific measures act counteracting each single cutaneous manifestation and they include both topical and systemic treatments depending on the severity of skin toxicities.

The patient should be informed and educated to recognize and immediately report any evidence of skin toxicity in order to promptly treat them and to ensure better outcomes [44].

Skin Rash

The management of the skin rash depends on the severity scored according to NCI CTCAE v4.0.

- Grade 1 (mild, poorly symptomatic, few lesions are identified). The suspension or the dose reduction of the EGFR inhibitor is not necessary in these patients, and only general measures are recommended [40, 44].
- Grade 2 (moderate, the rash is symptomatic, lesions are numerically higher than Grade1). As for Grade 1, the withdrawal or the dose reduction of the EGFR-inhibitor is not necessary. Topical antibiotics (clindamycin 1% gel, erythromycin 3% cream, metronidazole 0.75-1%) are suggested until the rash does not reach grade 1. If the scalp is involved, erythromycin 2% lotion may be prescribed.[40, 44]

When papular lesions predominate, systemic therapy is not recommended; conversely, in case of pustular elements, semisynthetic tetracyclines (minocycline 100 mg/day, doxycycline 100 mg/day) can be used for 4 weeks or until the rash is symptomatic [44].

In fact, tetracyclines are proved effective in reducing the severity of the skin rash through their imunomodulatory and anti-inflammatory properties; furthermore, they are able to suppress lymphocytes' proliferation, to inhibit neutrophils' migration and chemotaxis, inducing an over-expression of anti-inflammatory cytokines and reducing the synthesis of IL-6 [45].

Data on literature have reported the use of minocycline as preventive for the onset of the rash, despite there not statistically significant evidence that justify it [45-47].

Although several studies have demonstrated the efficacy of hydrocortisone 1% cream, topical corticosteroids are contraindicated in the treatment of the skin rash, as they promote microbial infection, and predispose to the development of steroid-related rosacea, atrophy and telangiectasia [20, 44].

Other studies have emphasized the efficacy of topical immunomodulators, such as calcineurin inhibitors tacrolimus (Protopic) and pimecrolimus (Elidel®), in the treatment of skin rash [45, 46].

Anti-acne treatments, as topical retinoids (adapalene, tazarotene) or benzoyl peroxide lotions and gels, are not indicated because they can cause irritation and dry skin [40].

The use of systemic steroids is not recommended as it may exacerbate the papular-pustular lesions and may hinder the mechanism of action of EGFR-Is [40].

- Grade 3 (severe, symptomatic, with a significant impact in patient's quality of life). The withdrawal of the treatment is recommended for a period of about 21 days or until the improvement of the rash to a degree 2. Once the improvement occurs, EGFR-Is can be restarted at the dose of 250 mg/m2; if any improvement is shown, the drug discontinuation is necessary. In case of a second or third recurrence of the skin rash, it is suggested to keep the reduced dose of EGFR-Is, whereas the definitive drug discontinuation is necessary if a fourth recurrence happens [5,40].

Topical treatments are the same of those used for grade 2, although a systemic therapy with semi-synthetic tetracycline and oral corticosteroids (methylprednisolone 0.4 mg/kg prednisone 0.5 mg/kg) for 10 days is necessary.

If the rash is highly symptomatic or non-responsive to treatments, oral retinoids (isotretinoin 0.3-0.5 mg/kg), corticosteroids iv (methylprednisolone, desamethasone), antihistamines im/iv (chlorphenamine), antibiotics iv (amoxicillin/clavulanic acid, gentamicin) and/or general hydration are recommended [40, 48, 49].

- Grade 4 (very severe, with significant impact on patient's the quality of life). Immediate discontinuation of EGFR-Is is mandatory. The topical and systemic measures are similar to those in Grade 2-3 [40].

If the papulo-pustular eruption is complicated by secondary infections, targeted antimicrobial treatment is prescribed. Any purulent collections should be incised and drained, in order to prevent sepsis.

New Therapeutic Options

The recent wide use of targeted cancer therapies have led to the development of new therapeutic strategies to effectively counter the dermatological toxicity associated with their use.

Vitamin K1, nicotinamide and green tea polyphenols have been identified as new potential therapeutic options in the treatment of the papulo-pustular rash.

A recent study have shown the efficacy of a cream containing urea and vitamin K1 0,1% (Reconval K1®): twice a day application of the cream has proven effective in reducing the frequency and intensity of the rash and in modulating the EGFR pathway without interfere with the anticancer treatment [50, 51].

In patients affected by Grade 1 skin rash, the application of the above cream has appeared useful to control cutaneous manifestation, whereas in patients affected by Grade 2 skin rash, the combined use of vitamin K1 and topical clindamycin 1% has been suggested [50, 51].

A further therapeutic option is the topical application of vitamin K3, also known as menadione, a water-soluble biosynthetic derivate vitamin K2 [41].

It is known that vitamin K3 is a potent inhibitor of phosphatases able to remove phosphate groups from different biological substrates, as EGFR. During EGFR-Is therapy, vitamin K3 reversibly inhibits the enzyme responsible for EGFR dephosphorylation, favoring an increased expression of the phosphorylated form, which is the metabolically active variant. Although no clinical studies have been conducted on this topic, preliminary data have emphasized an increased expression of the activated form of EGFR and an inhibition of phosphatase activity in mice receiving Erlotinib or Cetuximab and treated with menadione [52].

Nicotinamide (niacinamide or vitamin PP) belongs to vitamin B group and it is a component of the NAD (nicotinamide adenine dinucleotide) coenzyme. Nicotinamide has antioxidant, anti-inflammatory and immunomodulatory properties, inhibiting poly-ADP ribose polymerase I (PARP-I), an enzyme contributing to DNA repair. PARP-I increases the nuclear factor NF-kB-mediated transcription, which plays a central role in the expression of cytokines, adhesion molecules and inflammatory mediators [54, 55].

Nicotinamide also inhibits the expression of the adhesion molecule ICAM-I, of the major histocompatibility complex MHC class II, as well as the production of IL-12, IL-1 and TNF-α. Furthermore, it is a potent inhibitor of phosphodiesterase (PDE), increasing cyclic AMP, which, in turn, inhibits the proteases' release from leukocytes. Finally, the vitamin PP is able to remove reactive oxygen species (ROS) [54, 55].

In vitro studies have shown that nicotinamide is able to inhibit the IL-8 production through the inhibition of the phosphorylation of MAPK and NF-kB pathways, leading to the down-regulation of the NF-kB activity [55].

As concerns the skin rash, nicotinamide may act as anti-inflammatory and immunomodulator regulating MAPK pathway.

The green tea polyphenols are divided into:

- flavan-3-ols (catechins and their isomers
- flavandiols, flavonoids, phenolic acids (including gallic acid and its esters)
- Tannins [56]

Numerous studies have shown that polyphenols are endowed of anti-inflammatory, anti-oxidant properties and they are able to repair DNA damage UV-mediated [56].

We have recently demonstrated the efficacy of a combination therapy with systemic nicotinamide and topical green tea polyphenols cream in the management of skin rash induced by EGFR inhibitors [57].

This combined therapeutic approach resulted effective in papulo-pustular rash significantly improving itching and DLQI with a positive important psychological aspect in treated patients [57].

Conversely, this combination therapy was less effective in the treatment of paronychia, fissures and hair abnormalities [57].

Xerosis

Preventive measures and general daily use of emollients are the mainstay in the management of the xerosis associated to EGFR inhibitors.

The use of topical corticosteroids (betamethasone dipropionate 0.05%, flucinolone acetonide or hydrocortisone butyrate 0.1%) for 1-2 weeks is necessary when localized or diffuse erythema has been established.

Similarly, the use of topical antibiotics (fusidic acid 2%, bacitracin cream, mupirocin cream 2%) is recommended if there are yellow crusts due to secondary infection.

If eczema and/or desquamation are classified as Grade 3, the use of systemic steroids represent a useful therapeutic option to prevent the evolution to Grade 4.

Itching is the typical symptom associated to cutaneous xerosis and it should be managed either with urea-based emollients or with H1 antihistamines (cetirizine, loratadine, fexofenadine and ebastine) [16, 40, 58].

Fissures

The fissures can be treated with occlusive hydrocolloid dressings, with antiseptic solutions (potassium permanganate 0.025%) or topical applications of silver nitrate solutions, in order to favor the healing [16].

Perilesional area should be treated with urea-based emollients to promote healing and to prevent the flare-up [15].

Paronychia

In order to prevent paronychia, tight shoes should be avoided to reduce the pressure and friction. The paronychia should be treated daily with antiseptic solution (boric acid 3%) to prevent bacterial infection and ointments containing corticosteroids and antibiotics (gentamicin betamethasone 0.1% + 0.1% cream, betamethasone valerate 0.1% + 2% fusidic acid cream).

If infection is diffuse and/or severe, oral antibiotics (amoxicillin/ lavulanate, cephalexin, clindamycin) are needed, whereas oral analgesics are necessary if the patient complains pain.

Pyogenic granuloma-like lesions can be cauterized with silver nitrate or cryotherapy or dyatermocoagulation; surgical procedures are necessary only in selected cases [5, 16, 40].

References

[1] Seymour LK. Epidermal Growth Factor Receptor as a target: recent developments in search for effective new anti-cancer agents. *Curr. Drug Targets* 2001; 2: 117-133.

[2] Mendelson J. Targeting the Epidermal Growth Factor Receptor for cancer therapy. *J. Clin. Oncol.* 2002; 20: 1s-13s (Suppl 18).

[3] Ciardiello F, Tortora G. A novel approach in the treatment of cancer: targeting the Epidermal Growth Factor Receptor. *Clin. Cancer Res* 2001; 7: 2958-2070.

[4] Hu JC, Sadeghi P, Pinter-Brown L.C, Yashar S, Chiu M.V. Cutaneus side effects of Epidermal Growth Factor Receptor Inhibitors: clinical

presentation, pathogenesis and management. *J. Am. Acad. Dermatol.* 2007; 56: 317-326.

[5] Segaert S, van Cutsem E. Clinical signs, pathophysiology and management of skin toxicity during therapy with epidermal growth factor receptor inhibitors. *Ann. Oncol.* 2005, 16: 1425-1433.

[6] Wollenberg A, Moosmann N, Klein E and K. Katzer. A tool for scoring of acneiform skin eruptions induced by EGF receptor inhibition. *Exp. Dermatol.* 2008, 17: 790-792.

[7] Lacouture ME. Mechanism of cutaneous toxicities to EGFR inhibitors. *Nature Reviews Cancer*, 2006;6 (10):803-12.

[8] Lacouture ME, Maitland ML, Segaert S. A proposed EGFR inhibitor dermatologic adverse event-specific grading scale from the MASCC skin toxicity study group. *Support Care Cancer* 2010; 18:509-522.

[9] Lacouture ME, Basti S, Patel J, Benson A 3rd. The SERIES clinic. An interdisciplinary approach to the management of toxicities of EGFR inhibitors. *J. Support Oncol.* 2006; 4: 236-238.

[10] Newmann M, Gerami P, Guitart J et al. Histological differentiation of skin toxicity between cetuximab, erlotinib and panitumumab (single ErB1) and lapatinib (dual ErB1/2) epidermal growth factor receptor inhibitors. ASCO 2009. *J. Clin. Oncol.* 2009 (suppl).

[11] Jacot W, Bessis D, Jorda E, Ychou M, Fabbro M, Pujol JL, Guillot B. Acneiform eruption induced by epidermal growth factor receptor inhibitors in patients with solid tumours. *Br. J. Dermatol* 2004; 151(1):238–241.

[12] Ho C, Sangha R, Beckett L, Tanaka M, Lau DH, Eisen DB, Burich RA, Luciw P, Khan I, Mack PC, Gandara DR, Davies AM. Escalating weekly doses of cetuximab and correlation with skin toxicity: a phase I study. *Invest New Drugs* 2011; 29 (4): 680-7.

[13] Bianchini D, Jayanth A, Chua YJ, Cunningham D. Epidermal growth factor inhibitor-related skin toxicity: mechanisms, treatment and its potential role as a predictive marker. *Clin. Colorectal Canc.* (2008); 7: 33-43.

[14] Kimyai-Asadi A, Mh Jih. Follicular toxic effects of chimeric anti-epidermal growth factor receptor antibody cetuximab used to treat human and solid tumors. *Arch Dermatol* 2002; 138: 129-131.

[15] Segaert S, Chirtescu G, Lemmens L, Dumon K, Van Cutsem E, Tejpar S. Skin toxicities of targeted therapies. *Eur. J. Cancer* 2009; 45 (Suppl 1): 295-308.

[16] Lacouture ME, Laabs SM, Koehler M, Weetman RW, Preston AJ, Di Leo A, Gomez HL, Salazar VM, Byrne JA, Koch KM, Blackwell KL.. Analysis of dermatologic events in patients with cancer treated with lapatinib. Breast Cancer Res Treat 2009; 114: 485–493.

[17] Tsimboukis S, Merikas I, Karapanagiotou EM, WasifSaif M, Syrigos KM. Erlotinib- induced skin rash in patients with Non- Small-Cell lung cancer: pathogenesis, clinical significance, and management. *Clinical Lung Cancer* 2009; 10(2): 106-111.

[18] Busam KJ, Capodieci P, Motzer P, Kiehn T, Phelan D, Halpern AC. Cutaneous side- effects in patients treated with the antiepidermal growth factor receptor antibody C225. *Br. J. Dermatol* 2001; 144:1169-1176.

[19] Lynch TJ, Kim JR S, Eaby B, Garey J, West DP, Lacouture ME. Epidermal Growth Factor Receptor Inhibitor-Associated Cutaneous Toxicities: An Evolving Paradigm in Clinical Management. *The Oncologist* 2007; 12: 610-621.

[20] Galimont-Collen AFS, Vos LE, Lavrijsen APM. Classification and management of skin, hair, nail and mucosal side-effects of epidermal growth factor receptor (EGFR) inhibitors. *Eur. J. Cancer* 2007; 43: 845-851.

[21] Fernandez- Galar M, A. Espana, JM Lopez-Picazo. Acneiform lesions secondary to ZD1839, an inhibitor of the epidermal growth factor. *Clin. Exp. Dermatol.* 2004; 29: 138-140.

[22] Fox LP. Nail toxicity associated whit epidermal growth factor receptor inhibitor therapy. *J. Am. Acad. Dermatol.* 2007; 56: 460-465.

[23] Chang GC, Yang TY, Chen KC, Yin MC, Wang RC, Lin YC. Complications of therapy in cancer patients: case 1: Paronychia and skin hyperpigmentation induced by gefitinib in advanced non -small-lung cancer. *J. Clin. Oncol.* 2004; 22: 4646-8.

[24] Harris M. Monoclonal antibodies as therapeutic agents for cancer. *Lancet Oncol*. 2004; 5: 292-302.

[25] Ciardiello F, Bianco R, Damiano V, Fontanini G, Caputo R, Pomatico G, De Placido S, Bianco AR, Mendelsohn J, Tortora G. Antiangiogenic and antitumor activity of anti-epidermal growth factor receptor C225 monoclonal antibody in combination with vascular endothelial growth factor antisense oligonucleotide in human GEO colon cancer cells. *Clin. Cancer Res*. 2000; 6: 3739-47.

[26] Chanprapaph K, Vachiramon V, Rattanakaemakorn P. Epidermal growth factor receptor inhibitors: a review of cutaneous adverse events and management. *Dermatol. Res. Pract.* 2014;2014:734249.

[27] Osio A, Mateus C, Soria JC, Massard C, Malka D, Boige V, Besse B, Robert C. Cutaneous side-effects in patients on long-term treatment with epidermal growth factor receptor inhibitors. *Br. J. Dermatol* 2009; 161(3):515–521.

[28] Miettinem PJ, Berger JE, Meneses J, Phung Y, Pedersen RA, Werb Z, Derynck R. Epithelial immaturity and multiorgan failure in mice lacking epidermal growth factor receptor. *Nature* 1995; 376: 337-4.

[29] Philpott MP, Kaeley T. Effects of EGF on the morphology and patterns of DNA synthesis in isolated human hair follicles. *J. Invest Dermatol* 1994; 102: 186-91.

[30] Rodriguez NA, Ascaso FJ. Trichomegaly and poliosis of the eyelashes during Cetuximab treatment of metastatic colorectal cancer. *JCO* (2011); 29 (18): e532-533.

[31] Cohen PR, Escudier SM, Kurzrock R. Cetuximab associated elongation of the eyelashes: case report and review of eyelash trichomegaly secondary to Epidermal Growth Factor Receptor Inhibitors. *Am. J. Clin. Dermatol.* 2011; 12(1): 63-67.

[32] Donovan JC, Ghazarian DM, Shaw JC. Scarring alopecia associated with use of the epidermal growth factor receptor inhibitor gefitinib. *Archives of Dermatology*, vol. 144, no. 11, pp. 1524–1525, 2008.

[33] Graves JE, Jones BF, Lind AC, Heffernan MP. Non scarring inflammatory alopecia associated with the epidermal growth factor receptor inhibitor gefitinib. *J. Am. Acad. Dermatol.* 2006; 55(2); 349–353.

[34] Agero ALC, Dusza SW, Benvenuto-Andrade S, Busam KJ, Myskowski P, Halpern AC. Dermatologic side effects associated whit the epidermal growth factor receptor inhibitors. *J. Am. Acad. Dermatol.* 2006; 55: 657-670.

[35] Li T, Perez-Soler R. Skin toxicities associated with epidermal growth factor receptor inhibitors. *Targ Oncology* 2009; 4 (2): 107-119.

[36] Luu M, La S, Patel J, Guitart J, Lacouture ME. Photosensitive rash due to the epidermal growth factor receptor inhibitor erlotinib. *Photodermatol Photoimmunol Photomed* 2007; 23: 42-45.

[37] Jost M, FP Gasparro, PJ Jensen et al. Keratinocyte apoptosis induced by ultraviolet B radiation and CD95 ligation-differential protection through epidermal growth factor receptor activation and Bcl-x (L) expression. *J. Invest Dermatol.* 2001;116: 860-6.

[38] Li T, Perez-Soler R. Skin toxicities associated with epidermal growth factor receptor inhibitors. *Targ Oncology* 2009; 4 (2): 107-119.

[39] Sibaud V, Boralevi F, Vigarios E, Fricain JC. Oral toxicity of targeted anticancer therapies. *Ann. Dermatol. Venereol.* 2014;141(5):354-63.

[40] [40] Pinto C, Barone CA, Girolomoni G, Russi EG, Merlano MC, Ferrari D, Maiello E; American Society of Clinical Oncology; European Society of Medical Oncology. Management of skin toxicity associated with cetuximab treatment in combination with chemotherapy or radiotherapy. *Oncologist* 2011;16(2):228-38.

[41] Potthoff K, R Hofheinz, JC Hassel, Volkenandt M, Lordick F, Hartmann JT, Karthaus M, Riess H, Lipp HP, Hauschild A, Trarbach T, Wollenberg A. Interdisciplinary managent of EGFR-inhibitor-induced skin reactions: a German expert opinion. *Ann. Oncol.* 2011;22(3):524-35.

[42] Ouwerkerk J, Boers-Doets C. Best practices in the management of toxicities related to anti-EGFR agents for metastatic colorectal cancer *Eur. J. Oncol Nurs* 2010; 14: 337-349.

[43] Lacouture ME, Anadkat MJ, Bensadoun RJ, Bryce J, Chan A, Epstein JB, Eaby-Sandy B, Murphy BA; MASCC Skin Toxicity Study Group. Clinical practice guidelines for the prevention and treatment of EGFR inhibitor-associated dermatologic toxicities. *Support Care Cancer.* 2011;19(8):1079-95.

[44] Segaert S. Management of skin toxicity of epidermal growth factor receptor inhibitors. *Targ. Oncology* 2009; 3 245-25.

[45] Elling E, Brandt M, Schwartz T. Pimecrolimus: a novel treatment for cetuximab-induced papulopustolar eruption. *Arch. Dermatol.* 2008; 144: 1236-1238.

[46] Lynch TJ, Kim Jr S, Eaby B, Garey J, West DP, Lacouture ME. Epidermal Growth Factor Receptor Inhibitor-Associated Cutaneous Toxicities: An Evolving Paradigm in Clinical Management. *Oncologist* 2007; 12: 610-621.

[47] Scope A, Agero AL, Dusza SW,Myskowski PL, Lieb JA, Saltz L, Kemeny NE, Halpern AC. Randomized double-blind trial of prophylactic Oral Minocycline and topical tazarotene for cetuximab-associated acne like eruption. *J. Clin. Oncol.* 2007; 25(34): 5390-5396.

[48] Gutzmer R, Werfel T, Mao R, Kapp A, Elsner J. Successful treatment with oral isotretinoin of acneiform skin lesions associated with cetuximab therapy. *Br. J. Dermatol* 2005; 153 (4):849–851.

[49] Balagula Y, Garbe C, Myskowski P, Hauschild A, RapoportB,Boers-Doets CB, Lacouture ME. Clinical presentation and management of

dermatological toxicities of epidermal growth factor receptor inhibitors. *Int. J. Dermatol* 2011; 50:129–146.

[50] Ocvirk J. Management of cetuximab-induced skin toxicity with the prophylactic use of topical vitamin K1 cream. *Radiol. Oncol* 2010;44(4):265-6.

[51] Ocvirk J, Rebersek M. Topical application of vitamin K1 cream for Cetuximab-related skin toxicities. *Ann. Oncol.* 2009; 20 (7): VII 22-23.

[52] Perez-Soler R, Zou Y, Li T, Ling YH. The phosphatase inhibitor menadione (Vitamin K3) protects cells from EGFR inhibition by Erlotinib and Cetuximab. *Clin. Cancer Res.* 2011.

[53] Otte N, C Borelli, Korting HC. Nicotinamide-biologic actions of an emerging cosmetic ingredient. *Int. J. Cosmetic. Sci.* 2005; 27 (5):255-261.

[54] Namazi MR. Nicotinamide in dermatology: a capsule summary. *Int. J. Dermatol.* 2007; 46(12):1229-31.

[55] Grange PA, Raingeaud J, Calvez J, Dupin N. Nicotinamide inhibits Propionibacterium acnes-induced IL-8 production in keratinocytes though the NF-kB and MAPK pathways. *J. Dermatol Sci* 2009;56(2):106-12.

[56] Nichols Joi A, Santosh K. et al. Skin photoprotection by natural polyphenols: Anti-inflammatory, anti-oxidant and DNA repair mechanisms. *Arch. Dermatol. Res.* 2010; 302(2):71.

[57] Campanati A, Berardi R, Onofri A, Pierantoni C, Conte I, Giuliodori K, Molinelli E, Marcucci F, Cascinu S, Offidani A. A novel approach to manage skin toxicity caused by therapeutic agents targeting epidermal growth factor receptor. *Ann. Oncol.* 2012;23(4):1081-2.

[58] Rhee J, Oishi K, Garey J. Management of rash and other toxicities in patients treated with epidermal growth factor receptor-target agents. *Clin. Colorectal Cancer* 2005; 5 (suppl 2): S101-S106.

[59] Laabs SM, Koehler M, et al. Analysis of dermatologic events in patients with cancer treated with lapatinib. *Breast Cancer Res Treat* 2009; 114: 485–493.

In: New Skin Toxicities …
Editors: Giulia Ganzetti et al.
ISBN: 978-1-63482-224-4

Chapter 3

Skin Toxicities from VEGF Inhibitors

E. Molinelli*, MD and A. Offidani, MD, Professor
Dermatology Unit, Department of Clinical and Molecular Sciences,
Polytechnic Marche University, Italy

Abstract

The inhibition of the vascular endothelial growth factor receptor (VEGFR) represent an important step in the treatment of many neoplasms.

As for EGFR inhibitors, VGFR inhibitors are associated with cutaneous adverse effects that tend to increase patient's morbidity and influence patient's quality of life.

The incidence of cutaneous adverse events varies considerably by drug.

This manuscript aims to emphasize the skin toxicity associated with VEGFR inhibitors, focusing particularly on clinical presentation, pathogenetic mechanism, and therapeutic options.

* Corresponding author: molinelli.elisa@gmail.com.

The role of vascular endothelial growth factor (VEGF) signalling pathway in tumor angiogenesis has been extensively investigated and anti-angiogenic agents have emerged as an important therapeutic option for the treatment of advanced breast cancer, colorectal cancer, non-small cell lung cancer, hepatocellular and renal cell carcinoma. Dermatological side effects are relatively common among patients treated with VEGF inhibitors, particularly with receptor tyrosine kinase inhibitors (TKIs). (Table 1)

Table 1. Cutaneous and mucosal side effects of anti-angiogenic therapies

Bevacizumab	Sorafenib	Sunitinib
Mucosal bleeding-Hemorrhages	Hand-foot skin reaction	Hand-foot skin reaction
Stomatitis	Facial erythema	Skin discoloration
Disturbed wound healing	Subungual splinter hemorrhages	Papulopustular eruption
Thromboembolism	Alopecia	Hair depigmentation
Maculopapular rash	Stomatitis	Alopecia
	Xerosis	Subungual splinter hemorrhages
	Exanthematous eruption	Xerosis
	Skin cancer (SCC, KA)	Exanthematous eruption
	Eruptive melanocytic lesion	Edema

Monoclonal Antibodies against VEGF

Bevacizumab (Avastin®)

The most documented adverse events related to bevacizumab are mucosal bleeding and hemorrhages, oral mucositis, altered wound healing, and maculopapular eruptions [1, 2].

Oral toxicities include stomatitis, occurring in up to 10% of patients receiving bevacizumab; it is dose-independent and it is characterized by generalized erythema and sensitivity, and rarely by ulcers [3, 4].

The exact pathogenesis of mucositis is unclear; it has been hypothesized that bevacizumab could enhance the release of pro-inflammatory cytokines within the vascular endothelium, leading to mucosal irritation and ulceration [5].

Geographic tongue, a benign condition characterized by circinate or serpiginous, irregular, well-demarcated, erythematous, patchy erosions in bevacizumab-treated patients is also encountered [6]

Bevacizumab is also associated with increased risk of both arterial thromboembolic events (ATE) and venous thromboembolic events (VTE), which could involve cutaneous vasculature. Recently, a case of cutaneous thrombogenic vasculopathy associated with bevacizumab therapy has been described [7]

Notably, angiogenesis is an essential component of wound healing; altered or delay wound healing process in the surgical setting has been observed in bevacizumab-treated patients [8, 9]

As EGFR-inhibitors (EGFR-Is), bevacizumab causes cutaneous eruption, although they appear less frequent and severe. Non-specific skin rash showing as exfoliative dermatitis, hand eruption, and papular erythematous eruption involving the forehead, chest and back, have been described particularly in patients receiving bevacizumab and concomitant conventional chemotherapy [10-12] Moreover, perforating dermatosis and cutaneous lupus erythematosus have been reported [13, 14]

Acneiform eruptions affecting the face, upper trunk, and back have also been reported [15, 16]

As EGFRIs-associated skin toxicity, the incidence and severity of popular-pustular rash seems to positively correlate with treatment response and prognosis [16, 17].

Although the pathogenesis of acneiform eruption remains unknown, it has recently been demonstrated that VEGF regulates the proliferation and differentiation of both keratinocytes and follicular cells [18].

Thus, it is has been proposed that bevacizumab-related skin rash associated and EGFR-Is acneiform eruption may share similar pathogenic mechanism [16].

Lastly, localized skin necrosis of steroid-induced striae distensae has been described in bevacizumab-treated patient [19].

Recommendations for the Prevention and Management of Bevacizumab-Related Cutaneous Reactions

The prevention and treatment of cutaneous reactions are essential to improve the patients'quality of life and to avoid dose modifications that may affect treatment outcome. Primarily, any patient with signs and symptoms of skin or mucosal hemorrhages, thromboembolism or impaired wound healing, or within 28 days before and after major surgery, should not started bevacizumab treatment [20].

Symptomatic stomatitis can be ameliorated with antiseptic mouthwash (chlorexidine gluconate, diluite hydrogen peroxide), and aphthous ulcerations can be managed with topical steroids [1].

As papular-pustular rash following bevacizumab is very similar to EGFR-Is one, treatment could be comparable. Thus, topical antibiotics (clindamycin, erythromycin), systemic antibiotics (minocycline, doxycycline, tetracycline), short-term topical steroids (hydrocortisone, betamethasone dipropionate), and systemic steroids could be empirically used, according to the grade and duration of skin reaction. In addition, patients should avoid sun exposure, using physical photo-protection and sunscreen with a sun protection factor (SPF) of at least 30. Skin irritants should be avoided, particularly those containing alcohol and exfoliating agents, as topical anti-acne medications; suitable mild cleansing gel and hydrating moisturizer should be preferred [21].

VEGF Receptor Multi-Tyrosine Kinase Inhibitors

Dermatologic toxicities are among the most commonly reported adverse events in patients receiving treatment with sorafenib and sunitinib. The cutaneous toxicities associated with MKIs inhibitors include hand-foot skin reaction (HSFR), oral complications, hair and cutaneous pigmentary changes, and papulopustular rash. Xerosis, subungual hemorrhages, and exanthematous eruption are less frequently reported.

Sorafenib (Nexavar ®)

The most characteristic cutaneous adverse event is hand-foot skin reaction (HSFR), occurring in 10-62% of sorafenib-treated patients [22].

HSFR typically presents with palmo-plantar focal hyperkeratosis overlying an erythematous and edematous base, particularly affecting friction and trauma prone-areas, as the hell, lateral aspects of the soles, and interdigital spaces [23] (Figure 13).

HSFR is usually preceded or accompanied by palmo-plantar dysesthesia that begins as tingling and progress to burning sensation and pain, associated with an intolerance to contact with hot objects [24].

The erythema can evolve into blistering formation with subsequent desquamation, erosion, and ulceration [25].

Lesions usually manifest during the first 2-4 weeks of treatment and symptoms recur with repeated doses of MKI [26].

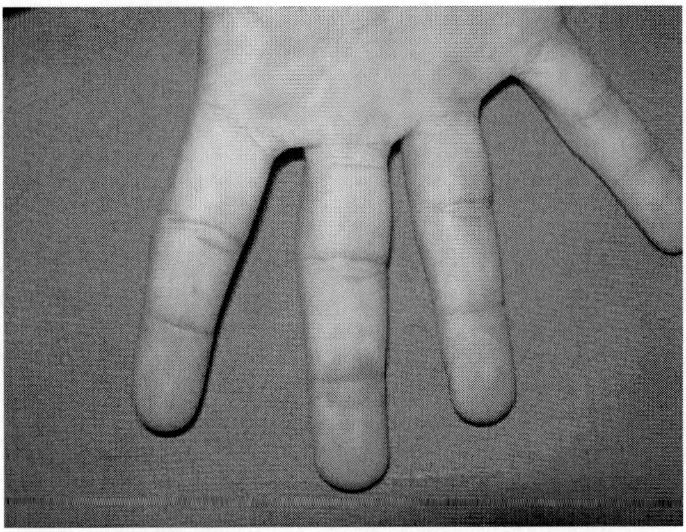

Figure 13.

Additionally, HSFR may also involve the dorsal surfaces of the hands and feet and may develop into painful erythematous plaques involving non-acral areas, as face, inguinal, and flexures areas or pressure sites [1].

Hand-foot syndrome (HSF), also known as acral erythema or palmo-plantar erythrodysesthesia, is a well-documented adverse effect of a wide range of conventional chemotherapeutic agents, as capecitabine, 5-fluorouracil, cytarabine, docetaxel, and pegylated liposomal doxorubicin [27].

HSF has a distinctive clinical presentation, characterized by symmetric, sharply, demarcated erythematous plaques on the palms and soles, predominantly located on the later aspect of the fingers and distal fat pads [28].

In contrast to classic HSF, HSFR is generally more localized and hyperkeratotic, affecting the soles more than palms, particularly the friction-prone areas [29].

Histologically, HSFR is characterized by prominent acanthosis with hyperkeratosis, dermal edema, and perivascular cell infiltrate, mostly composed of lymphocytes [24, 30]. Immunohistochemistry demonstrates cytokeratin 10 loss and concomitant increased expression of cytokeratin 14, suggesting that sorafenib may inhibit keratinocyte differentiation [30] (Table 2).

Table 2. Hand-foot syndrome and Hand-foot skin reaction

	HFS **Hand-foot syndrome**	**HFSR** **Hand-foot skin reaction**
Causative agents	Pegylated liposomal doxorubicin, capecitabine, 5-fluoruracil, cytarabine, docetaxel, doxorubicin	Multikinase inhibitors (sorafenib, sunitinib, axitinib, pazopanib, regorafenib)
Risk factors	Dosage, female gender	Tumour type (RCC), female gender, liver metastases, affected organ number
Sites involved	Palms more than soles, dorsal hands and feet	Soles more than palms Pressure-bearing areas (fingertips, interdigital web spaces, heals, lateral aspect of the feet, over joints)
Clinical features	Symmetric erythema and edema in palms and soles	Localized hyperkeratosis overlying an erythematous base
Histopathology	Basal layer vacuolar degeneration, spongiosis, hyperkeratosis, parakeratosis	No vacuolar degeneration, well-defined band of discohesive dyskeratotic keratinocytes

Although the diagnosis of HSFR is principally clinical, differential diagnosis may be considered, including graft-versus-host diseases, erythema multiforme, contact dermatitis, vasculitis, erythromelalgia, and other drug reactions [30].

The pathogenesis of HFSR remains largely unknown: it is thought to be a direct toxic effect of MKIs given the dose dependency demonstrated in sorafenib-treated patients [31].

As HSF, HFSR appears to be secondary to accumulation in the eccrine ducts and excretion in the sweet of antiangiogenic agents. The predilection of HSFR for the palms and soles may be a consequence of the high concentration of eccrine sweet gland in these areas [28].

However, the sorafenib excretion in sweat has not been proven, making this hypothesis unlikely with HFSR and multi-kinase inhibitors [1, 25].

Notably, sorafenib and sunitinib are potent inhibitors of VEGFR, PDGFR, c-KIT, Fms-like tyrosine kinase 3 (Flt-3), and RET. The simultaneous inhibition MKIs-related of VEGFR and PDGFR that mediate repair process could hypothetically exacerbate localized tissue damage and inflammation, particularly in the sites predisposed to microtrauma, as the extremities [28].

In addition, HSFR is rarely observed when the aforementioned receptors are individually inhibited, and in antiangiogenic agents that specifically target VEGFR [1].

Moreover, VEGFR inhibition appears to have a crucial role in HFSR pathogenesis; this is evidenced by a higher HFSR incidence in patients receiving combined anti-angiogenic therapy with sorafenib and bevacizumab [32]. Individual genetic variability could also influence the risk of HFSR [28].

Interestingly, tumor type may influence MKI-induced HFSR; sorafenib-treated patients with renal cell carcinoma exhibiting higher rates of HFSR compared with patients affecting by other malignancies. Additional risk factors are female gender, liver metastases and affected organs number [30].

Lastly, HSFR is currently considered a marker of tumor response and of favourable clinical outcomes in patients receiving sorafenib [33].

Facial erythema resembling to seborrheic dermatitis has been described in 63% of patients treated with sorafenib. It usually occurs within the first weeks of treatment and spontaneously resolves after MKI discontinuation. Scalp dysesthesia may precede or accompanied the skin manifestation [23, 25]. The underlying mechanism is largely unknown; available evidence suggests that the inhibition of RAF, rather than VEGF or PDGFR, may be implicated in the erythema onset [34].

Splinter subungual hemorrhages have been noted in 70% of patients receiving sorafenib. Clinically, they manifest as single or multiple linear black or brown streaks under the fingernails, less frequently the toenails. Subungual hemorrhages present during the first 2 months of therapy and resolve without treatment. The antiangiogenic effect of sorafenib may play a role in splinter hemorrhages formation [1].

Alopecia occurs in up to 27% of patients taking sorafenib, and it is characterized by thinning, patchy hair loss and slow beard growth. It usually develops approximately 3-15 weeks after treatment initiation, and it is reversible after cessation of medication [24]. In addition, patients treated with sorafenib have exhibited hair abnormalities, as curlier, finer, and brittler hair on the scalp and extremities. Interestingly, a significant correlation between occurrence of alopecia and severity of HFSR has been described [1]. (Figure14)

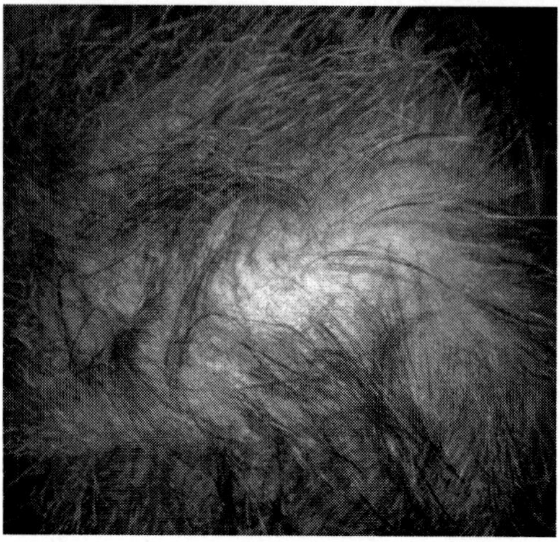

Figure 14.

Mild to moderate stomatitis has been reported in 26% of patients receiving sorafenib. Generally, oral lesions appear early and it is not dose-related. As alopecia, it directly correlates to the severity of HFSR [25].

Pruritus and xerosis have been documented in up to 10% of sorafenib-treated patients. Xerosis, typically presents as dry, scaly, itchy skin, primarily affecting the lower limbs [35]. The itching may also be independent from skin dryness, appearing early and involving mainly the scalp. The pathogenesis is probably related to excretion of drug metabolites through the sudoriparous glands, which are highly diffuse in the scalp [36] (Figure 15).

Exanthematous eruptions, reminiscent hypersensitivity drug reactions, have been noted in 20% of patients receiving sorafenib [1].

Importantly, sorafenib therapy has been associated with increase susceptibility to premalignant and malignant skin lesions, including actinic keratosis (AK), keratoacanthomas (KAs), and squamous cell carcinomas (SCC) [37]. Peculiarly, within few months sorafenib-treated patients can develop cutaneous neoplasms in non-photodamaged skin and without previous history of malignant skin lesions [38]. Occasionally, AK and KAs spontaneously regress after sorafenib discontinuation; a decrease in size and number of lesions upon MKI cessation, followed by a rapid increase in lesions size or number, after restarting the medication have also been observed [39].

Several theories have been proposed to explain the relationship between sorafenib and skin cancers. It has been postulated that the development of sorafenib-induced SCC may be related to RAF inhibition, resulting in the paradoxical activation of MAPK signalling in the context of mutated or activated RAS keratinocytes and favouring epithelial proliferation [40].
Eruptive melanocytic lesion in patients receiving sorafenib has also been reported, although the exact percentage is unknown; no reported cases of melanoma have been noted [41].

Other cutaneous side effects associated with sorafenib treatment are generalized keratosis pilaris-like eruption, nipple hyperkeratosis, and epidermal cysts. Single reports of erythema multiform-like eruption and localized dyskeratotic plaque with milia are also reported [22].

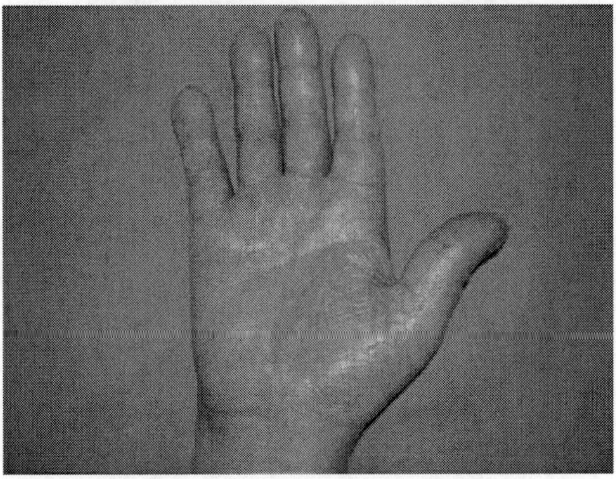

Figure 15.

Sunitinib (Sutent ®)

Similar to sorafenib, hand-foot skin reaction (HSFR) is observed in patients receiving sunitinib, occurring in 10% to 28% of patients and clinically presenting as painful symmetric erythematous plaques of the palms and soles. In addition, skin yellowish discoloration, hypo- or depigmentation has been reported in 28% of patients receiving sunitinib. It usually involves the face, with sparing of the sclera and mucosa. The pigmentation may be caused by the deposition of sunitinib metabolites which contain a yellow/orange powder. The discoloration occurs within a few weeks of treatment and it is reversible with drug discontinuation [22].

Approximately 10% and 6% of patients manifest hair depigmentation and alopecia, respectively. The hair depigmentation or greying usually occurs after 5-6 weeks of treatment. It is a dose-dependent phenomenon; the alternating areas of depigmented and pigmented hair is analogous to the treatment cycles and confirm these hypothesis. The pathogenesis of hair changes is related to the inhibition of c-Kit, which are involved in melanin synthesis. Additionally, a yellow discoloration of the hair has been observed in about 30% of patients [1].

Papulo-pustular rash similar to seborrheic-dermatitis-like eruption and interesting the face, upper chest, and back, have been described in association to sunitinib treatment [34] (Figure 16).

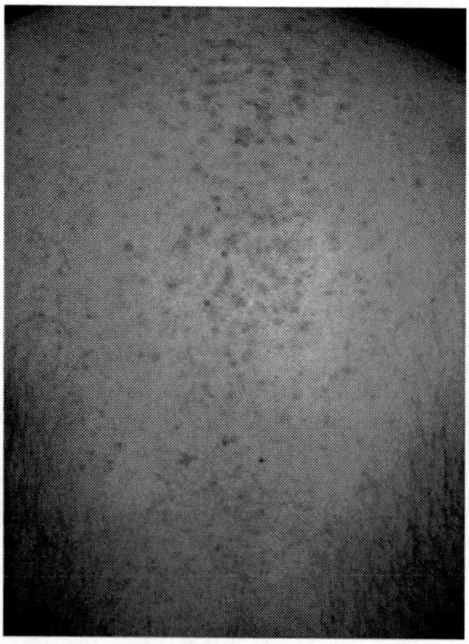

Figure 16.

Sunitinib can also produce dose-dependent exanthematous eruptions that typically presents as maculopapular exanthemas and affect 40% of patients [20].

Interestingly, periorbital and occipital oedema has been reported in up to 50% of patients receiving sunitinib [23].

It has been postulated that facial edema may be caused by the inhibition of PDGFR that mediates vascular permeability and increases dermal interstitial fluid, leading to fluid retention [22].

Moreover, patients receiving sunitinib are particularly prone to developing xerosis and subungual hemorrhages, as sorafenib-treated patients. Phototoxicity has rarely been described among patients receiving sunitinib treatment [1].

Severity Grading System

The ability to accurately assess and grade dermatological toxicities is critical as treatment strategy vary based on the severity of muco-cutaneous adverse events. Skin toxicities associated to antiangiogenic agents have been categorized by the National Cancer Institute Common Terminology Criteria Adverse Events (NCI-CTCAE) version 4.0 [42] (Table 3).

Table 3. NCI-CTCAE version 4.0 toxicity scale for adverse events associated with VEGF inhibitors: dermatologic adverse events

Adverse event	Grade	Clinical manifestations
Maculopapular rash	1	Macules/papules covering < 10% BSA with or without symptoms (e.g., pruritus, burning, tightness)
	2	Macules/papules covering 10-30% BSA with or without symptoms (e.g., pruritus, burning, tightness), limiting instrumental ADL
	3	Macules/papules covering > 30% BSA with or without symptoms (e.g., pruritus, burning, tightness), limiting self-care ADL
Papulopustular/acneiform rash	1	Papules and/or pustules covering < 10% BSA, which may or may not be associated with symptoms of pruritus or tenderness
	2	Papules and/or pustules covering 10-30% BSA, which may or may not be associated with symptoms of pruritus or tenderness, associated with psychosocial impact, limiting instrumental ADL

Table 3. (Continued)

Adverse event	Grade	Clinical manifestations
Papulopustular/acneiform rash (continued)	3	Papules and/or pustules covering >30% BSA, which may or may not be associated with symptoms of pruritus or tenderness, limiting self-care ADL, associated with local superinfection, with oral antibiotics indicated
	4	Papules and/or pustules covering any BSA, which may or may not be associated with symptoms of pruritus or tenderness and are associated with associated with extensive superinfection, with IV antibiotics indicated, with life-threating consequences
	5	Death
Hand-foot skin reaction	1	Minimal skin changes or dermatitis (e.g., erythema) without pain
	2	Skin changes (e.g., peeling, blisters, edema or hyperkeratosis) with pain, limiting instrumental ADL
	3	Severe skin changes (e.g., peeling, blisters, edema or hyperkeratosis) with pain, limiting self-care
Pruritus	1	Mild or localized topical intervention indicated
	2	Intense or widespread, intermittent skin changes from scratching (e.g., edema, excoriations, lichenification, oozing/crusts); oral interventions indicated, limiting instrumental ADL
	3	Intense or widespread, constant, limiting self-care ADL or sleep, oral corticosteroid or immunosuppressive therapy indicated
Alopecia	1	Hair loss <50% of normal for that is not obvious from a distance but only on close inspection, a different hair style may be required to cover the hair loss but it does not require a wig or a hair piece to camouflage
	2	Hair loss ≥ 50% of normal for that individual that is readily apparent to others, a wig or hair piece is necessary if the patients desires to completely camouflage the hair loss, associated to psychosocial impact

Adverse event	Grade	Clinical manifestations
Mucositis	1	Asymptomatic or mild symptoms, intervention not indicated
	2	Moderate pain, not interfering with oral intake, modified diet indicated
	3	Severe pain, interfering with oral intake
	4	Life-threating consequences, urgent intervention indicated
	5	Death

Recommendations for the Prevention and Management of MKIs-Related Cutaneous Reactions

The management of MKIs-related cutaneous reactions, including HFSR, represents a great challenge for both oncologist and dermatologist. Clinical data derived from prospective and placebo-controlled randomized trials are few and they remain the main limitation of the current available treatments [43].

Patient's education is crucial in therapeutic management, and life-style modifications, as the use of a thick alcohol-free emollient to moisturize dry skin, warm water and avoidance of prolonged, hot shower to minimize the xerosis, are recommended [43].

Concerning HFSR, preventive measures are central to treatment strategy and include reducing exposure of hands and feet to hot water, avoiding rubbing and vigorous exercises, and exfoliating hyperkeratotic lesions. High-potency topical corticosteroids to decrease inflammation may be helpful. Supportive measures also comprise wound care for erosions and ulcerations, topical keratolytics (urea-based cream) to decrease hyperkeratosis, and frequent emollient use [44].

Recently, it has been demonstrated the efficacy of topical heparin in the treatment of HFS, reducing skin inflammation, dosing interruption, and MKI discontinuation [45].

Generally, severe reactions may require a dose reduction (grade 2) or delaying (grade 3) MKIs treatment, for a minimum of one week. When treatment is restarted, the dose should be decreased; if the grade 3 symptoms recur for the third time, sorafenib or sunitinib should be discontinued [29, 46].

Dryness and pruritus have a large impact on quality of life. Gentle skin care using cool or lukewarm baths, mild soap, fragrance- and alcohol-free emollients are advised. Systemic antihistamines, pregabalin, and gabapentin may be useful to reduce itchiness. In addition, patients should be warned to limit sun exposure [22].

Exanthematous eruptions may require antihistamines and topical or oral steroids; dose reductions or treatment interruptions are not required [1].

Management of skin cancer includes cryotherapy of AK and conventional excision of KAs or SCC; watchful waiting in the case of KAs since spontaneous regression may occur. Close dermatologic follow-up are advised. The interruption of MKI treatment is not required [38].

The papulopustular rash can be treated with topical or systemic antibiotics, as acneiform eruption EGFRIs-related [1].

Importantly, skin discoloration, subungual hemorrhages, and hair changes should not limit MIKs therapy [22].

Novel Antiangiogenic Agents and Cutaneous Side Effects

Several antiangiogenic agents targeting VEGF are recently approved for the treatment of diverse progressive and metastatic malignancies. In addition, the development of novel targeted therapies contributes to improve our understanding of tumorigenesis. Aflibercept (Zaltrap®) is a recombinant fusion protein interacting with VEGF-A and VEGF-B isoforms, indicates, in combination with 5-fluorouracil, for patients with metastatic colorectal cancer [47]. The most common adverse reactions with aflibercept include hand-foot skin reaction (HSFR), hyperpigmentation changes, and altered wound healing, though not much literature is yet available on aflibercept cutaneous side effects [48].

Skin hyperpigmentation aflibercept-associated may be managed with depigmenting agents, as hydroquinone 4%, azelaic acid 15%, and avoiding sun exposure [47].

In addition, novel upcoming multi-kinase inhibitors will presumably extend the therapeutic armamentarium over the coming years. Pazopanib (Votrient®), cediranib (Recentin®), vandetanib (Zactima®), regorafenib (Stivarga®), and axitinib (Inlyta®) can inhibit several serine-threonine and receptor kinases, including VEGFR. As sorafenib and sunitinib, they cause HFSR, stomatitis, thromboembolic events, maculopapular eruption, bleeding, and hair depigmentation, especially pazopanib-treated patients. In addition, pazopanib seems to be associated with a lower risk of HFSR than the aforementioned agents [1].

Future studies assessing the dermatologic reactions related to antiangiogenic inhibitors, particularly in combination to conventional chemotherapeutic drugs, are mandatory.

References

[1] Ishak, RS; Aad, SA; Kyei, A; Farhat, FS. Cutaneous manifestations of anti-angiogenic therapy in oncology: Review with focus on VEGF inhibitors. *Crit Rev Oncol Hematol*, 2014, 90(2), 152-64.

[2] Gressett, SM; Shah, SR. Intricacies of bevacizumab-induced toxicities and their management. *Ann Pharmacother*, 2009, 43(3), 490-501.

[3] Glade Bender, JL; Adamson, PC; Reid, JM; Xu, L; Baruchel, S; Shaked, Y; Kerbel, RS; Cooney-Qualter, EM; Stempak, D; Chen, HX; Nelson, MD; Krailo, MD; Ingle, AM; Blaney, SM; Kandel, JJ; Yamashiro, DJ. Phase I trial and pharmacokinetic study of bevacizumab in pediatric patients with refractory solid tumors: a Children's Oncology Group Study. *J Clin Oncol*, 2008, 26(3), 399-405.

[4] Cohen, MH; Gootenberg, J; Keegan, P; Pazdur, R. FDA drug approval summary: bevacizumab plus FOLFOX4 as second-line treatment of colorectal cancer. *Oncologist*, 2007, 12(3), 356-61.

[5] Watters, AL; Epstein, JB; Agulnik, M. Oral complications of targeted cancer therapies: a narrative literature review. *Oral Oncol*, 2011, 47(6), 441-8.

[6] Gavrilovic, IT; Balagula, Y; Rosen, AC; Ramaswamy, V; Dickler, MN; Dunkel, IJ; Lacouture, ME. Characteristics of Oral Mucosal Events Related to Bevacizumab Treatment. *Oncologist*, 2012, 17(2), 274-8.

[7] Kiuru, M; Schwartz, M; Magro, C. Cutaneous thrombogenic vasculopathy associated with bevacizumab therapy. *Dermatol Online J*, 2014, Jun 15, 20(6).

[8] Scappaticci, FA; Fehrenbacher, L; Cartwright, T; Hainsworth, JD; Heim, W; Berlin, J; Kabbinavar, F; Novotny, W; Sarkar, S; Hurwitz, H. Surgical wound healing complications in metastatic colorectal cancer patients treated with bevacizumab. *J Surg Oncol*, 2005, 91(3), 173-80.

[9] Cohen, RB; Oudard, S. Antiangiogenic therapy for advanced renal cell carcinoma: management of treatment-related toxicities. *Invest New Drugs*, 2012, 30(5), 2066-79.

[10] Kabbinavar, F; Hurwitz, HI; Fehrenbacher, L; Meropol, NJ; Novotny, WF; Lieberman, G; Griffing, S; Bergsland, E. Phase II, randomized trial

comparing bevacizumab plus fluorouracil (FU)/leucovorin (LV) with FU/LV alone in patients with metastatic colorectal cancer. *J Clin Oncol*, 2003, 21(1), 60-5.

[11] Ruiz, V; Garcia-Muret, MP; Alomar, A. Hand eruption after intravenous administration of bevacizumab. *J Eur Acad Dermatol Venereol*, 2011, 25(2), 238-9.

[12] Saif, MW; Longo, WL; Israel, G. Correlation between rash and a positive drug response associated with bevacizumab in a patient with advanced colorectal cancer. *Clin Colorectal Cancer*, 2008, 7(2), 144-8.

[13] Vano-Galvan, S; Moreno, C; Medina, J; Pérez-García, B; García-López, JL; Jaén, P. Perforating dermatosis in a patient receiving bevacizumab. *J Eur Acad Dermatol Venereol*, 2009, 23(8), 972-4.

[14] Vihinen, P; Paija, O; Kivisaari, A; Koulu, L; Aho, H. Cutaneous lupus erythematosus after treatment with paclitaxel and bevacizumab for metastatic breast cancer: a case report. *J Med Case Rep*, 2011, 5, 243.

[15] Gotlib, V; Khaled, S; Lapko, I; et al. Skin rash secondary to bevacizumab in a patient with advanced colorectal cancer and relation to response. *Anticancer Drugs*, 2006, 17, 1227-1229.

[16] Keenan, BP; Abuav, R. Acneiform eruption in a patient receiving bevacizumab for glioblastoma multiforme. *Arch Dermatol*, 2010, 146(5), 577.

[17] Gavrilova, M; Martin, JM; Martin-Gorgojo, A; Jorda-Cuevas, E. Follicular acneiform eruption induced by bevacizumab. *Dermatol Online J*, 2012, 18(9), 15.

[18] Man, XY; Yang, XH; Cai, SQ; et al. Expression and localization of vascular endothelial growth factor and vascular endothelial growth factor receptor-2 in human epidermal appendages: a comparison study by immunofluorescence. *Clin Exp Dermatol*, 2009, 34, 396-401.

[19] Fourcade, S; Gaudy-Marqucste, C; Tasei, AM; Richard, MA; Grob, JJ. Localized skin necrosis of steroid-induced striae distensae: an unusual complication of bevacizumab and irinotecan therapy. *Arch Dermatol*, 2011, 147(10), 1227-8.

[20] Wozel, G; Sticherling, M; Schön, MP. Cutaneous side effects of inhibition of VEGF signal transduction. *J Dtsch Dermatol Ges*, 2010, 8(4), 243-9.

[21] Peuvrel, L; Dréno, B. Dermatological toxicity associated with targeted therapies in cancer: optimal management. *Am J Clin Dermatol*, 2014, 15(5), 425-44.

[22] Reyes-Habito, CM; Roh, EK. Cutaneous reactions to chemotherapeutic drugs and targeted therapy for cancer: Part II. Targeted therapy. *J Am Acad Dermatol*, 2014, 71(2), 217.e1-217.e11.

[23] McLellan, B; Kerr, H. Cutaneous toxicities of the multikinase inhibitors sorafenib and sunitinib. *Dermatol Ther*, 2011, 24(4), 396-400.

[24] Autier, J; Escudier, B; Wechsler, J; Spatz, A; Robert, C. Prospective study of the cutaneous adverse effects of sorafenib, a novel multikinase inhibitor. *Arch Dermatol*, 2008, 144(7), 886-92.

[25] Lee, WJ; Lee, JL; Chang, SE; Lee, MW; Kang, YK; Choi, JH; Moon, KC; Koh, JK. Cutaneous adverse effects in patients treated with the multitargeted kinase inhibitors sorafenib and sunitinib. *Br J Dermatol*, 2009, 161(5), 1045-51.

[26] Lacouture, ME; Reilly, LM; Gerami, P; Guitart, J. Hand foot skin reaction in cancer patients treated with the multikinase inhibitors sorafenib and sunitinib. *Ann Oncol*, 2008, 19(11), 1955-61.

[27] Reyes-Habito, CM; Roh, EK. Cutaneous reactions to chemotherapeutic drugs and targeted therapy for cancer: Part I. Targeted therapy. *J Am Acad Dermatol*, 2014, 71(2), 203.e1-203.e12.

[28] Miller, KK; Gorcey, L; McLellan, BN. Chemotherapy-induced hand-foot syndrome and nail changes: a review of clinical presentation, etiology, pathogenesis, and management. *J Am Acad Dermatol*, 2014, 71(4), 787-94.

[29] Robert, C; Mateus, C; Spatz, A; Wechsler, J; Escudier, B. Dermatologic symptoms associated with the multikinase inhibitor sorafenib. *J Am Acad Dermatol*, 2009, 60(2), 299-305.

[30] Lipworth, AD; Robert, C; Zhu, AX. Hand-foot syndrome (hand-foot skin reaction, palmar-plantar erythrodysesthesia): focus on sorafenib and sunitinib. *Oncology*, 2009, 77(5), 257-71

[31] Fischer, A; Wu, S; Ho, AL; Lacouture ME. The risk of hand-foot skin reaction to axitinib, a novel VEGF inhibitor: a systematic review of literature and meta-analysis. *Invest New Drugs*, 2013, 31(3), 787-97.

[32] Azad, NS; Posadas, EM; Kwitkowski, VE; Steinberg, SM; Jain, L; Annunziata, CM; Minasian, L; Sarosy, G; Kotz, HL; Premkumar, A; Cao, L; McNally, D; Chow, C; Chen, HX; Wright, JJ; Figg, WD; Kohn, EC. Combination targeted therapy with sorafenib and bevacizumab results in enhanced toxicity and antitumor activity. *J Clin Oncol*, 2008, 26(22), 3709-14.

[33] Jain, L; Sissung, TM; Danesi, R; Kohn, EC; Dahut, WL; Kummar, S; Venzon, D; Liewehr, D; English, BC; Baum, CE; Yarchoan, R;

Giaccone, G; Venitz, J; Price, DK; Figg, WD. Hypertension and hand-foot skin reactions related to VEGFR2 genotype and improved clinical outcome following bevacizumab and sorafenib. *J Exp Clin Cancer Res*, 2010, 29:95.

[34] Robert, C; Soria, JC; Spatz, A; Le Cesne, A; Malka, D; Pautier, P; Wechsler, J; Lhomme, C; Escudier, B; Boige, V; Armand, JP; Le Chevalier, T. Cutaneous side-effects of kinase inhibitors and blocking antibodies. *Lancet Oncol*, 2005, 6(7), 491-500.

[35] Ensslin, CJ; Rosen, AC; Wu, S; Lacouture, ME. Pruritus in patients treated with targeted cancer therapies: systematic review and meta-analysis. *J Am Acad Dermatol*, 2013, 69(5), 708-20.

[36] Bracarda, S; Ruggeri, EM; Monti, M; Merlano, M; D'Angelo, A; Ferraù, F; Cortesi, E; Santoro, A; Sorafenib Working Group. Early detection, prevention and management of cutaneous adverse events due to sorafenib: recommendations from the Sorafenib Working Group. *Crit Rev Oncol Hematol*, 2012, 82(3), 378-86.

[37] Arnault, JP; Wechsler, J; Escudier, B; Spatz, A; Tomasic, G; Sibaud, V; Aractingi, S; Grange, JD; Poirier-Colame, V; Malka, D; Soria, JC; Mateus, C; Robert, C. Keratoacanthomas and squamous cell carcinomas in patients receiving sorafenib. *J Clin Oncol*, 2009, 27(23), e59-61.

[38] Williams, VL; Cohen, PR; Stewart, DJ. Sorafenib-induced premalignant and malignant skin lesions. *Int J Dermatol*, 2011, 50(4), 396-402.

[39] Kwon, EJ; Kish, LS; Jaworsky, C. The histologic spectrum of epithelial neoplasms induced by sorafenib. *J Am Acad Dermatol*, 2009, 61(3), 522-7.

[40] Oberholzer, PA; Kee, D; Dziunycz, P; Sucker, A; Kamsukom, N; Jones, R; Roden, C; Chalk, CJ; Ardlie, K; Palescandolo, E; Piris, A; MacConaill, LE; Robert, C; Hofbauer, GF; McArthur, GA; Schadendorf, D; Garraway, LA. RAS mutations are associated with the development of cutaneous squamous cell tumors in patients treated with RAF inhibitors. *J Clin Oncol*, 2012, 30(3), 316-21.

[41] Kong, HH; Sibaud, V; Chanco Turner, ML; Fojo, T; Hornyak, TJ; Chevreau, C. Sorafenib-induced eruptive melanocytic lesions. *Arch Dermatol*, 2008, 144(6), 820-2.

[42] National Cancer Institute. Common Terminology Criteria Adverse Events v4.0. NCI, NHI, DHHS. May, 29, 2009 NHI publication.

[43] Lacouture, ME; Wu, S; Robert, C; Atkins, MB; Kong, HH; Guitart, J; Garbe, C; Hauschild, A; Puzanov, I; Alexandrescu, DT; Anderson, RT; Wood, L; Dutcher, JP. Evolving strategies for the management of hand-

foot skin reaction associated with the multitargeted kinase inhibitors sorafenib and sunitinib. *Oncologist*, 2008, 13(9), 1001-11.

[44] Belum, VR; Cercek, A; Sanz-Motilva, V; Lacouture, ME. Dermatologic adverse events to targeted therapies in lower GI cancers: clinical presentation and management. *Curr Treat Options Oncol*. 2013, 14(3), 389-404.

[45] Li, JR; Yang, CR; Cheng, CL; Ho, HC; Chiu, KY; Su, CK; Chen, WM; Wang, SS; Chen, CS; Yang, CK; Ou, YC. Efficacy of a protocol including heparin ointment for treatment of multikinase inhibitor-induced hand-foot skin reactions. *Support Care Cancer*, 2013, 21(3), 907-11.

[46] Rosenbaum, SE; Wu, S; Newman, MA; West, DP; Kuzel, T; Lacouture, ME. Dermatological reactions to the multitargeted tyrosine kinase inhibitor sunitinib. *Support Care Cancer*, 2008, 16(6), 557-66.

[47] Ruff, P; Ferry, DR; Lakomý, R; Prausová, J; Van Hazel, GA; Hoff, PM; Cunningham, D; Arnold, D; Schmoll, HJ; Moiseyenko, VM1; McKendrick, JJ; Ten Tije, AJ; Vishwanath, RL; Bhargava, P; Chevalier, S; Macarulla, T; Van Cutsem, E. Time course of safety and efficacy of aflibercept in combination with FOLFIRI in patients with metastatic colorectal cancer who progressed on previous oxaliplatin-based therapy. Eur J Cancer [Epub ahead of print].

[48] Belum, VR; Wu, S; Lacouture, ME. Risk of hand-foot skin reaction with the novel multikinase inhibitor regorafenib: a meta-analysis. *Invest New Drugs*, 2013, 31(4), 1078-86.

In: New Skin Toxicities ...
Editors: Giulia Ganzetti et al.
ISBN: 978-1-63482-224-4

Chapter 4

Skin Toxicity from BRAF Inhibitors

A. Campanati*[*]*, MD, and A. Offidani, MD, Professor
Dermatology Unit, Department of Clinical and Molecular Sciences,
Polytechnic Marche University, Italy

Abstract

In the last two years, a new era in the treatment options for patients with metastatic cutaneous melanoma has come. Targeted therapies with the inhibitors of the RAS-RAF-MEK-ERK pathway (BRAF inhibitors) have substantially changed the therapeutic management of advanced melanoma. These agents are able to induce remarkable results for patients, but at the same time they have introduced a therapeutic challenge in the field of melanoma, owing to drug resistance and their clinical toxicity, which represent the two most discussed issues. For Dermatologists, the most intriguing "off target" effects of these target therapies are cutaneous adverse reactions. The therapeutic management of skin toxicities is mandatory to improve patients' outcome and quality of life. Moreover it puts dermatologists in a never ever thought position in the therapy of advanced melanoma. This manuscript reports the state of the art of skin toxicity associated with BRAF inhibitors, focusing particularly on clinical presentation, histopathological findings, and specific therapeutic options.

[*] Correspondence to: anna.campanati@gmail.com.

The Mapk Pathway

There is now growing evidence that adverse events associated with RAF and / or MEK-inhibitors, are similar to those induced by EGFR-inhibitors [1]: acneiform eruptions, cutaneous xerosis, photosensibility, paronychia and hair changes [2, 3]. This is not surprising, since RAF and MEK both represent major downstream mediators of EGFR signaling. However, while clinical-histological extensive data on EGFR-inhibitors toxicity are present in literature, [4] data on MEK1/2 inhibitors are still lacking.

The intracellular mitogen-activated protein kinase (MAPK) pathway, also known as the 'Ras-RAF-MEK-ERK pathway', is a sequential enzyme cascade involving the activation of Ras, RAF, and MEK and ERK kinases sequentially. In the MAPK pathway, EGFR plays a crucial regulator role for epidermal homeostasis. Downstream of EGFR, Ras activation mediates survival, proliferation of keratinocytes, and inhibits their differentiation [5-7]. The interaction between Ras, RAF, and MEK and ERK kinases is based on classic feedback loop mechanisms consisting of upstream signals and inhibitory components. However, besides the well-known interaction between the major players of the MAPK pathway (RAS, RAF, MEK and ERK kinases, an intricate crosstalk with other poorly enunciated parallel signaling pathways within the cell and other extracellular factors complicate the full understood of the MAPK pathway.

Several receptor mutations, gene amplification, feedback loop elements' disruption and/ or increased autocrine or paracrine signaling could exert an influence on this pathway, leading to abnormal up-regulation of the MAPK pathway [8, 9].

The Raf/MEK/ERK cascade is probably the best-described Ras effector pathway: humans have three Raf isoforms (A-RAF, B-RAF and RAF-1 or C-RAF), all three RAF can be activated by Ras and phosphorylate MEK, B-RAF is the most effective and is necessary for ERK activation in vivo [10].

ERK stimulation leads to phosphorylation of transcription of several other factors, structural proteins and metabolic enzymes, promoting proliferation and inhibiting differentiation in the epidermis [11].

According to experimental data, the inhibition of the MAPK pathway in keratinocytes, either at the level of EGFR or at the level of MEK, results in keratinocyte cell death, decreased cell migration, and inflammation, which can cause dermatologic toxicity through different mechanisms [12]. Firstly, the skin barrier is compromised and the MEK–ERK-dependent induction of antimicrobial peptides, [13] blocked by the inhibition of EGFR signaling leads to an increase of secondary infections. Moreover the MAPK-dependent epithelial wound healing becomes suboptimal [14].

Beyond the cutaneous side effects, similar to those of EGFRI, recent findings suggest that RAF/MEK-inhibitors can be implicated in the development of borderline and malignant keratinocyte skin tumors such as keratoacanthomas and SCC [15]. This effect could be explained by the RAF inhibition inducing a paradoxical activation of the MAPK signaling pathway in those cells without BRAF mutation, resulting in an increased risk of skin epithelial tumors. Only a minority of treated patients develop skin tumors, thus if a preceding mutations or signaling deviations are required to induce this peculiar side effect of BRAF-inhibitors still remains uncleared [16]. Accordingly, based on the most recent molecular analyses in cutaneous squamous-cell carcinomas and keratoacanthomas of patients treated with vemurafenib, mutations in RAS seem to be frequent [17].

Genetic aberrations in the MAPK pathway are present in over 80% of cutaneous melanomas, including abnormalities in Ras, RAF, MEK and ERK [18-20]. The most common mutation appears to be in the BRAF, occurring in 36%–59% of primary melanomas and 42%–66% of metastatic melanomas [19-20] and has been characterized as an oncogenic mutation [21]. The most common somatic mutation is found at V600E in exon 15 in 66%–90% of BRAF mutant melanomas [22-25]. This is a point mutation in DNA (1799T-A) resulting in a single amino-acid substitution at Valine 600 to Glutamic acid in the activating segment, which leads to elevated kinase activity compared with BRAF wild type, stimulated phosphorylation of downstream endogenous ERK and subsequent cellular proliferation and survival [26, 27].

The V600K mutation has been reported in 7%–28.5% of patients with BRAF mutant metastatic melanoma [28-31] and involves two point mutations (GTG to AAG) with a lysine for valine substitution. Other non-V600E mutations have also been reported and will become increasingly relevant in interpretation of future clinical trials.

The presence of a BRAF mutation is a demonstrated poor prognostic factor with a strong association with worse outcome in the metastatic setting.

Braf Inhibitors

Preclinical data demonstrated that selective BRAF inhibition results in growth arrest and induction of apoptosis in cell lines and xenograft models [32,33].

Activating mutations of the BRAF oncogene are targets for the "selective", Class I, [vemurafenib, dabrafenib and "non-selective", Class II, (sorafenib) BRAF inhibitors. The first ones exert their action on the mutated form of BRAF kinases (producing constitutive oncogenic signaling), while the latter inhibits the resting conformation of the enzyme with minimal action against tumors with point mutations in V600EBRAF [34].

Vemurafenib received regulatory agency approval in 2011 for the treatment of patients with unresectable or metastatic melanoma carrying the V600E BRAF mutation [35], and dabrafenib is currently in Phase II/III clinical trials. Sorafenib is an oral multi-kinase inhibitor approved for treating advanced renal cell carcinoma [36, 37] and unresectable hepatocellular carcinoma [36, 38], regardless of the BRAF mutation status of the tumor. It did not demonstrated any successful for malignant melanoma carrying BRAF mutations In monotherapy regimen [39]. In addition to being a potent BRAF and CRAF kinase inhibitor, sorafenib also inhibits vascular endothelial growth factor receptors (VEGFR) -1, -2, and -3, platelet-derived growth factor receptor (PDGFR)-β, fms-like tyrosine kinase 3 (FLT-3), c-KIT, and RET receptor tyrosine kinases [40]. Thus, the sorafenib's activity stems from a combination of its anti-proliferative and pro-apoptotic effects, as well as its anti-angiogenic properties [37]. All the three BRAF inhibitors show similar ability to active paradoxically the MAPK pathway in normal keratinocytes, sharing the same risk to improve the incidence of several skin neoplasms.

Cutaneous Toxicity

The clinical spectrum of cutaneous toxicity to BRAF inhibitors seems to be dose and exposure dependent phenomenon [41]. Generally, skin manifestations could be classified in four sub-groups: inflammatory reactions, benign and proliferative skin lesions, pre-malignant and malignant skin lesions, and less common reactions.

Table 1. Skin Manifestations

Skin manifestations	**Therapeutic management**
I. INFLAMMATORY	
Rash (maculopapular, papular,folliculocentric, seborrheic-dermatitis-like)	Grade 1 – Topicals: cold compresses, moisturizing creams, topical cortison-like creams; topical steroid creams (e.g., hydrocortisone 1–2.5%, triamcinolone acetonide 0.025%, clobetasol propionate 0.05%), antibiotic creams (e.g., Clindamycin 1%, Metronidazole 0.75%) Grade 2/3 – Oral corticosteroids, oral antibiotics, low-dose acitretin; consider dose modification/ interruption of targeted therapy drug
Pruritus	Grade 1 – Topicals: cold compresses, wet dressings, moisturizing creams, topical cortison-like creams; topical steroid creams (e.g., hydrocortisone 1–2.5%, triamcinolone acetonide 0.025%, clobetasol propionate 0.05%), antibiotic creams (e.g., Clindamycin 1%, Metronidazole 0.75%) Grade 2 – Add oral antihistamines (benadryl, hydroxyzine) GABA agonists (gabapentin, pregabalin) Grade 3 – Consider addition of oral corticosteroids
Photosensitivity	Grade 1 – Topicals: moisturizers, topical cortison-like creams; steroids (hydrocortisone 2.5%, triamcinolone 0.1%) Grade 2/3 – Topicals: steroids (hydrocortisone 2.5%, triamcinolone 0.1%); Oral antihistamines or corticosteroids; pain control with NSAIDs Barrier: proper clothing, broad-rimmed hats, UVA/B sunscreen (SPF 50+) liberally, avoid sun exposure
Alopecia	Topical minoxidil 2–5% bid
Hand and Foot Skin Reaction	Prevention avoid friction, traumatic activity, constrictive footwear; use thick cotton gloves or socks; shoes with padded insoles Grade 1 – Topical: keratolytic moisturizing creams (urea 20–40%, salicylic acid 6%, ammonium lactate 12%) Grade 2 – Topical: keratolytic moisturizing creams (urea 20-40%, salicylic acid 6%, ammonium lactate 12%),topical high-potency steroids, topical anesthetic creams (lidocaine 3%, EMLA); oral: analgesics, NSAIDs, GABA agonists, opioids Grade 3 –consider dose reduction or temporary/permanent discontinuation of targeted therapy drug

Table 1. (Continued)

Skin manifestations	Therapeutic management
II. SQUAMOPROLIFERATIVE BENIGN LESIONS Skin papillomas Verrucous keratoses Viral warts Seborrheic keratoses (SK) Palmar/plantar hyperkeratosis	Physical: cryotherapy, electrocautery/fulguration, CO2 laser 2 Surgical: excision or shave removal (for larger lesions) Medical: Topical medications (podophyllotoxin 0.5% solution, imiquimod 5% cream, intralesional bleomycin) or topical keratolytic agents (e.g., 20–50% salicylic acid and urea)
III. SQUAMOPROLIFERATIVE PRENEOPLATIC AND NEOPLASTIC LESIONS Actinic keratoses (AK) Keratininzing tumours – KTS (Keratoacanthomas KA; Squamous cell carcinoma SCC, basal cell carcinoma BCC)	Multiple and eruptive lesions: watchful waiting policy, topical medications (imiquimod 5%), diclofenac 3%, physical therapies (electrocautery, PDT), oral therapies Ingenol mebutate (acitretin, bexarotene). Dose reduction or therapy interruption Full-body skin examinations before starting therapy and every 2 months during therapy Counseling and education on photoprotection (broadband sunscreens)
IV. MELANOCITIC LESIONS Nevi Melanoma	Referral to a dermatologist for evaluation and monitoring
IV. UNCOMMON REACTIONS Milia, acantholytic dyskeratosis, panniculitis-like lesions, and toxic erythema-like reactions	

I. Inflammatory Reactions

Rash

8-25% of patients receiving vemurafenib exhibit maculopapular rashes (Figure 17) [42, 43]. 10-66% of patients under sorafenib develop a folliculotropic rash (Figure 18) [44-46], and only 6% of dabrafenib treated patients develop grade 2 rash [47]. Rush usually appears after 2 weeks of treatment and it could be asymptomatic; lesions can involve face, neck and trunk and extremities [48], tends to be pleomorphic (papular, maculopapular, folliculotropic) and may be associated with occasional scaling. Lesion like Keratosis pilaris has been noted in 5–9% of patients on trials [42, 43].

The acneiform eruptions typical of EGFR inhibitors, have been only rarely reported [49].

It is noteworthy that even in cases of severe rashes induced by BRAF inhibitors re-challenge does not result in worsening or precipitation of life-threatening reactions [49]. Management includes gentle skin care, topical moisturizing and cortisol-like creams, topical or oral corticosteroids, topical or oral antibiotics, and dose reduction/interruption depending on the severity of skin toxicity (Table 1) [41]. Low-dose acitretin (10 mg) has demonstrated to be useful in a patient with facial follicular papules [50].

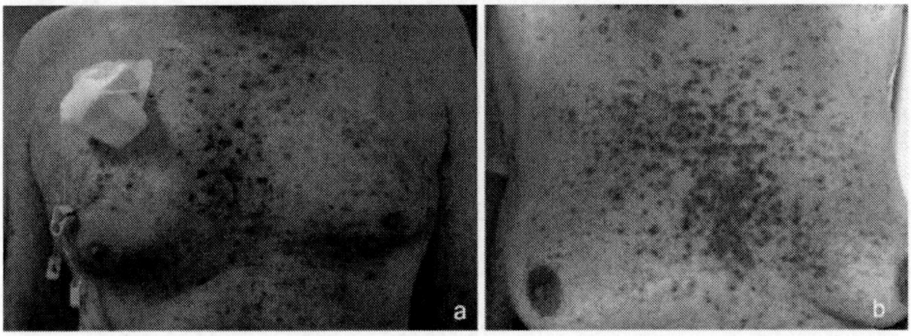

Figure 17. Maculo-papular rash in patients receiving vemurafenib a) and sorafenib b).

Pruritus

Pruritus can occur in up to 22–30% of patients treated with vemurafenib [42, 43], in 8-19% of patients receiving sorafenib, and it is usually mild (Figures 17-18) [44]. It has not been reported with dabrafenib yet.

Pruritus could be related to the xerosis and the inflammatory changes ok skin present in up to 16–19% and 23% of patients treated with vemurafenib [42, 43] and sorafenib [51]. Managing dry skin and rash may help to relieve patients from pruritus. It is recommended that patients avoid hot showers and fragranced soaps, decrease bathing time, use alcohol-free emollients to moisturize instead of lotions, and avoid ointments that may increase follicular occlusion [2]. For pruritus, cold compresses and wet dressings, along with topical moisturizing, cortisol-like creams, topical corticosteroids and topical cortison-like cream can be therapeutic for some patients, while patients with grades 2/3 pruritus (6–7% patients) may benefit from oral antihistamines, GABA agonist or oral steroids.

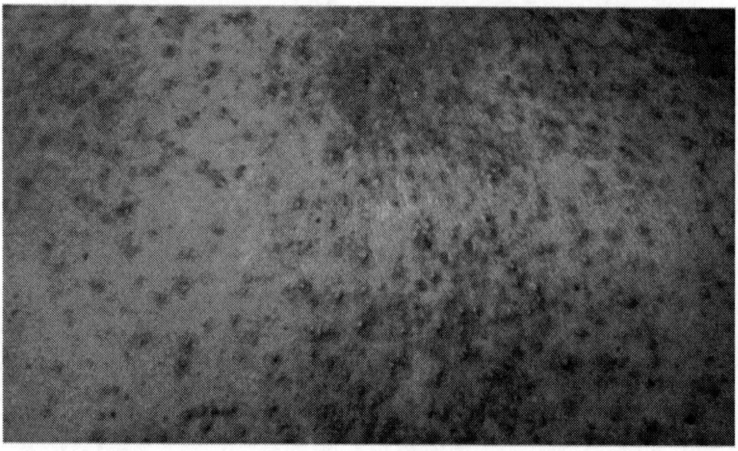

Figure 18. Folliculotropic rash in patiens receiving sorafenib.

Photosensitivity

Photosensitivity is the most common side effect, and it has been reported in 30–52% of vemurafenib-treated patients in Phase II/III clinical trials [42, 43]. Similar reactions with dabrafenib are rare [25]. The onset seems to be within 24 hours of sun exposure and usually in summer [49]. In Sun exposed area erythema and painful blistering, even with limited daily activities (e.g., driving), can occur. This is due to the UVA-dependent nature of the phototoxicity, which is known to penetrate glass [52].

Management strategies employed for other photosensitizing disorders in routine practice should be applied to these patients. They should be advised to use UVA/UVB-protective sunscreens (SPF 50+) liberally, using at least one fluid ounce to cover sun-exposed areas, and reapplying every 2 hours. They should wear appropriate clothing and hats, and develop routine habits to minimize possible UV exposure on both sunny and cloudy days.

Alopecia

Hair loss can occur with vemurafenib (36%) (Figure 19) [42, 42], dabrafenib (20%) [11], and sorafenib (27-53%) [31, 37]. Alopecia presents between the third and fifteenth weeks of treatment and may spontaneously resolve without interruption of therapy. It has a significant impact on patients' quality of life, as known. Scalp cooling and topical minoxidil 2% have shown some therapeutic benefit [16]. Although hair generally grows back following discontinuation of therapy, even if patients should be advised that they could become more brittle and curlier than before.

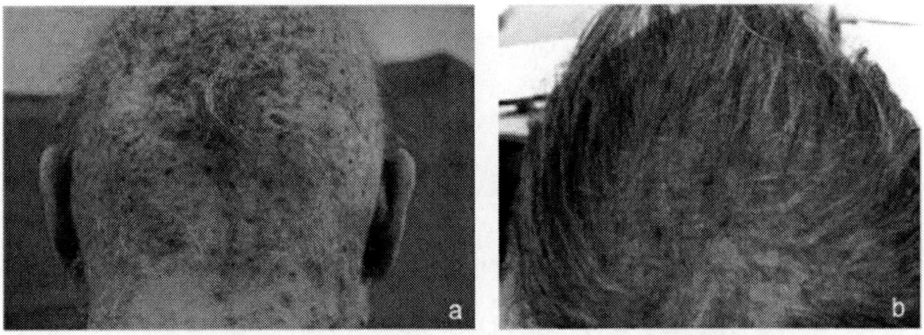

Figure 19. Diffuse alopecia in patient receivning vemurafenib a) and sorafenib b).

Hand Foot Skin Reaction (HFSR)

HFSR is considered the most specific dermatologic toxicity for patients receiving sorafenib, and it can occur in 9-34% of patients [53]. It presents with painful, tender, localized, erythematous lesions that classically on palms and soles, subjected to increased friction; sometimes lesions can involve toes (Figure 20). After some weeks, skin becomes blistering, thickened and hyperkeratotic, these symptoms can exert a great impact on patients' quality of life, interfering with their ability to perform daily activities [44]. HFSR could be the direct consequence of a dose-dependent, dual blockade of VEGF and PDGF receptors, which could lead into reduced ability to repair blood vessels damage in areas subjected to repeated and subclinical trauma [12].

However, also dabrafenib and vemurafenib have been related to HFSR also, [30, 31], thus a class action could be inferred for BRAF inhibitors to induce HFSR [22].

Therapeutic management of HFSR is based mainly on its prevention, since when the reaction is difficult to treat in sé.

Prevention includes early removing of hyperkeratotic areas of palms and soles, wearing soft shoes, cotton socks, orthotic shoes, and avoiding tight-fitting shoes, running, or any activity able to increase friction to palms and soles unnecessarily [16]. Treatment of HSFR reaction depends from its severity. Current recommendations include keratolytic moisturizers containing urea, salicylic acid, or ammonium lactate for grade 1 reactions, with added topical corticosteroids, and twice daily application of topical anesthetic creams (lidocaine, EMLA) for painful blisters of grade 2 events. Grade 3 toxicity often necessitates dose interruptions, and analgesics such as 2% lidocaine, non-steroidal anti- inflammatory drugs (NSAIDs), GABA agonists and opioids may help patients to relief from pain [16, 54].

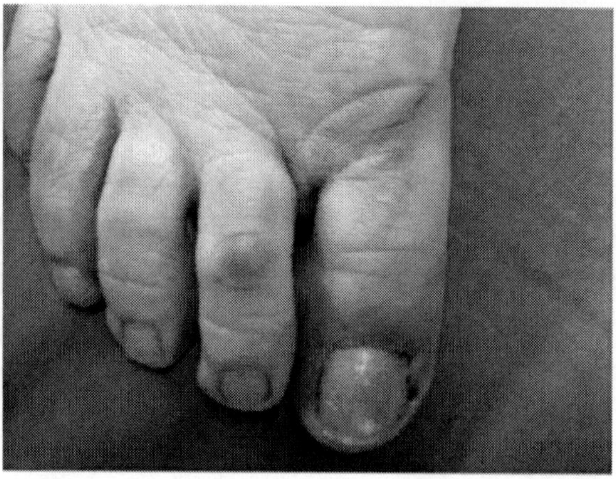

Figure 20. Hand Foot Skin Reaction in patient receinivn sorafenib. Particular of skin lesions in the toes.

2. Squamoproliferative Benign Lesions

Skin Papillomas

Approximately 18–30% of patients receiving vemurafenib develop papillomas [42, 43]; however, the clinical relevance for these skin reactions is not significant, and clear clinical descriptions of them or are still lacking.

Generally papillomas are benign, skin colored lesions usually arising from the neck and trunk. (common in the general population), and malignant degeneration has not been reported to this date.

Verrucous Keratoses

The onset of benign warty-like growing lesions without viral cytopathic changes or HPV infection occurred in 86% of patients receiving vemurafenib or dabrafenib [22].

These lesions resemble clinically viral warts, even if they are associated with a mild to severe atypia, not apparently related with the duration of treatment.

As progressive degrees of dysplasia were noted in these lesions, it could be inferred that these represent evolutionary stages of lesions from benign to malignant, and should be managed with excision or cryotherapy.

Viral Warts

Viral Warts occur commonly (30%) in vemurafenib-treated and dabrafenib-treated patients [30], and have been reported also in a minority of patients receiving sorafenib. managed with excision and cryotherapy [31]. The causative role of HPV, and which serotype are mainly involved in these patients have not been identified yet. Since vemurafenib does not seem to induce immunosuppression, the complex interplay between RAS activation, UV exposure, and prevalence of HPV on sun-exposed skin in the general population might be responsible for viral wart development [30].

These lesion can be easily managed though ablative methods (e.g., cryotherapy, lasers)

Seborrheic Keratoses (SKs) and Palmo-Plantar Hyperkeratosis

Seborrheic keratoses have been reported in 6–14%, of patients in Phase II/III trials with vemurafenib [42, 43] and in (34%) of patients under dabrafenib. Hyperkeratosis was observed in up to 19–28% of patients receiving vemurafenib and in 22–26% receiving dabrafenib [42, 43]. Treatment is usually based on physical ablation of lesions with cryotherapy or laser surgery.

3. Squamoproliferative Neoplastic and Preneoplastic Lesions: Actinic Keratosis - AK, Keratininzing Tumours - KTS (Keratoacantoma - KA, Squamous Cell Carcinoma - SCC, Basal Cell Carcinoma - BCC)

Keratinizing skin tumors (KTS) are one of the most intriguing and concerning side effects of BRAF target therapies, and dermatologist should be aware about this risk (Table 1). Patients may develop solitary or multiple lesions gradually or in an eruptive manner, and in various combinations of AKs, KAs, SCCs, and BCC (BCC) [11, 26, 31].

AK have been reported in 6-16% of patients receiving vemurafenib and in the (5–10%) of patients receiving dabrafrenib [42] and dabrafenib [11]. Also sorafenib is associated with the risk of development of AK., whose inflammatory features makes it at higher risk for evolution into SCC [16]. In sorafenib-treated patients AK sometimes resolve spontaneously after discontinuing treatment, and has a preference for previously sun-damaged skin, suggesting the hypothesis that these lesions could be inflamed pre-existing AKs [24].

Pre-existing lesions that can progress to squamous cell carcinomas at a 10% rate have been reported, but whether BRAF inhibition hastens their progression is not defined yet. However, prompt treatment with cryotherapy, topical imiquimod, photodymanimc therapy, ingenol mebutate is advised to prevent a potentially more rapid progression to SCC than in patients who have not received BRAF inhibitors [40].

Cutaneous SCCs and KAs have been reported in up to 4–31,<11%, and in 6–7% of patients receiving vemurafenib [42,48] dabrafenib [26, 27, 28, 39], and sorafenib [19], respectively. This however, may vary with trial duration, dosage and length of follow- up. They tend to appear early during the course of treatment (median time ~8 weeks) with vemurafenib [20], but may occur anytime from 1 to 9 months after initiating sorafenib treatment [19]. Notably, the face, neck, back, arms, and legs are commonly affected with vemurafenib, while one study in Australians reported that dabrafenib-induced SCCs developed predominantly on sites (67% on upper arm, chest, and/or thigh) different from those usually reported (head, neck, forearm, hand, and/or lower leg) [29]. Interestingly, one study on patients receiving sorafenib reported that all lesions developed at the expense of, or around, hair follicles, suggesting that follicular keratinocytes are particularly involved [19]. The presence of RAS mutations with a higher frequency in lesions on sun-exposed skin suggests that these agents could be not directly carcinogenic; rather they could potentiate preexisting oncogenic processes [40]. This might account for the higher incidence in older individuals and on photo- exposed sites [41]. Clinically, the lesions are fast growing, non-pigmented and dome-shaped nodules, with a central keratotic zone, and usually appear on histology as well-differentiated SCCs (KA-type or KA-like). The potential for blood and lymphatic invasion seems to be limited, and there have been no reports of perineural or metastatic spread [19, 20, 23]. Furthermore, the dose-reduction did not offset the appearance of new lesions, suggesting a dose-independent mechanism [30]. The activation of CRAF in wt-BRAF cells by a BRAF inhibitor could explain their occurrence [10–12]. RAS- activating mutations were found in SCCs and KAs in patients treated with vemurafenib and sorafenib, and lesions may also develop through RAF inhibitory mechanisms in the skin, specifically affecting follicular keratinocytes [19, 42, 43]. In general, several factors [environmental (UVR), genetic (e.g., EDV)] including mutations of p53/p16INK4 inhibitor/RAS, complicated molecular/ cytogenetic aberrations, and HPV have all been implicated in the development of SCCs [40, 44–46]. Whether similar, auxiliary or different mechanisms have a role in BRAF-inhibition induced SCCs remains uncleared.

Basal cell carcinomas have also been noted with vemurafenib and sorafenib, and are likely due to an activated MAP kinase pathway [30].

Management of cutaneous neoplasms in patients receiving these medications includes regular monitoring for development of squamoproliferative skin lesions. In addition, a thorough dermatological evaluation before initiation of therapy is highly recommended. When confronted with suspicious lesions, histopathological analysis is recommended, and physicians should have a low threshold for biopsy and treatment. Standard of care provides management (cryotherapy/simple excision), and dose modification or discontinuation is usually not required, as local treatment is generally sufficient [41]. However, if patients on sorafenib have multiple, unresectable lesions, or evidence of relapse post- treatment, clinicians may consider interrupting therapy, which may lead to spontaneous resolution of symptoms [47]. Interestingly, one study reported that when dabrafenib and trametinib (MEK inhibitor) were given in combination, SCCs did not develop, although benign keratoses appeared [23]. On the other hand, another clinical trial did not confirm that proliferative skin lesions were significantly reduced with combined BRAF and MEK inhibition [48]. Another recent report described the benefit of acitretin 25 mg in a patient with eruptive KAs [49]. Bexarotene, successful used for treatment of sorafenib-induced lesions [50], has not been used with vemurafenib or dabrafenib yet. There effective use of photodynamic therapy for treating multiple vemurafenib-associated KAs and SCCs is debated, and it could provide an appropriate non-invasive solution for managing patients receiving BRAF inhibitors [51]. Strict monitoring for KSTs is advised for up to 6 months after stopping the targeted therapy [13]. Finally, photo-protection appears protective.

4. Melanocytic Lesions

Although melanocitic proliferations are less common, this is one of the most concerning adverse events that mandates close monitoring and follow-up of patients receiving BRAF inhibitors. The underlying mechanistic concepts seem consistent with the experimental in vitro findings of paradoxical activation of wt-BRAF cells (via CRAF activation) when treated with BRAF inhibitors [10], supported by BRAF wild-type status of all new melanocytic lesions [52].

Activated nevi, regression, second primary melanomas and atypical melanocytic proliferations have been reported in patients treated with BRAF inhibitors [26, 52, 53]. In Phase II/III trials, malignant melanoma was noted in 3/336 [9] and 2/132 [21] patients, and melanocytic nevi were noted in 7/132 [21] patients. There are no reports of metastases to date. The benefit of combination therapies to avoid such events are being investigated [48].

There have also been a limited number of case reports of eruptive nevi and lentigines secondary to sorafenib therapy. Lesions may appear 1–24 months after initiating treatment, and have an acral predilection [54-56]. This lesions could result from the activated MAP kinase pathway in the skin. It is interest to report that nevi were not related to high sun exposure in patients [12].

Early detection of subtle changes in melanocytic lesions is paramount. Therefore, a long-term dermoscopic follow-up in all patients on BRAF inhibitors should be recommended [52, 53]. This is particularly relevant in sun- damaged skin and fair-skinned individuals. Close monitoring and prompt treatment is mandatory for continued use of these medications, since early lesions (even melanomas) are easily manageable, and timely management outweighs the associated risks of withholding lifesaving cancer treatment.

5. Less Common Reactions

Eruptive Milia

Eruptive milia are other less common sequelae of vemurafenib treatment [30, 41]. Similar lesions have been noted with dabrafenib and EGFR inhibitors (gefitinib, matuzumab) [29].

Acantholytic Dyskeratoses

Acantholytic dyskeratoses including Darier-like and Grover-like rashes (single/ multiple lesions) with supportive histopathology were seen in 8/14 of patients in one report [23].

Miscellaneous nonspecific lesions noted with dabrafenib treatment in individual patients were: pyogenic granuloma, abscess formation, lichen simplex, angiofibroma, angioma, eczema, dermatofibroma, itchy skin and vitiligo [29]. However, there was no causal relationship.

The accompanying cutaneous and systemic adverse events rarely necessitate dose interruption or discontinuation, and a minimal reduction, or in some cases a brief interruption, seems to suffice [9, 20]. Close and careful visual inspection, dermoscopy, and histopathology are important for establishing the diagnosis.

Panniculitis

Panniculitis-like subcutaneous lesions associated with arthralgias have been recently reported in patients on vemurafenib and dabrafenib [41]. The eruptions were associated with pain and necessitated brief interruption.

Toxic Erythema-Like Eruption

A toxic erythema-like eruption was reported in a case series of patients on vemurafenib. The drug did not trigger a hypersensitivity reaction upon restarting after dose-interruption, suggesting a possible upregulation of an alternate signaling pathway [41].

Conclusion

In recent years, the use of BRAF inhibitors has grown exponentially, causing the emergence of a wide spectrum of cutaneous toxicities. Among them, the development of secondary cutaneous malignancies appears to be the most intriguing and constant finding, and has received great attention.

Although such toxicities are not preventable, increasing evidence suggests that they follow a predictable pattern/course, and are manageable. There is, however, an urgent need for the development of evidence-based management strategies to effectively tackle such events.

A cross-disciplinary approach between oncologists and dermatologists is crucial to develop shared treatment protocols and optimize management.

References

[1] Gutzmer R, Becker JC, Enk A et al. Management of cutaneous side effects of EGFR inhibitors: recommendations from a German expert panel for the primary treating physician. *J Dtsch Dermatol Ges* 2011; 9: 195–203.

[2] Balagula Y, Lacouture ME, Cotliar JA. Dermatologic toxicities of targeted anticancer therapies. *J Support Oncol* 2010; 8: 149–161.

[3] Querfeld C, Duffy K, Magel G et al. Disseminated follicular eruption during therapy with the MEK-inhibitor AZD6244. *J Am Acad Dermatol* 2011; 64: e17–e19.

[4] Guttman-Yassky E, Mita A, De Jonge M et al. Characterisation of the cutaneous pathology in non-small cell lung cancer (NSCLC) patients treated with the EGFR tyrosine kinase inhibitor erlotinib. *Eur J Cancer* 2010; 46: 2010–2019.

[5] Khavari TA, Rinn J. Ras / Erk MAPK signaling in epidermal homeostasis and neoplasia. *Cell Cycle* 2007; 6: 2928–2931.

[6] Kern F, Niault T, Baccarini M. Ras and Raf pathways in epidermis development and carcinogenesis. *Br J Cancer* 2011; 104: 1240.

[7] Karnoub AE, Weinberg RA. Ras oncogenes: split personalities. *Nat Rev Mol Cell Biol* 2008; 9: 517–531.

[8] Downward J. Targeting RAS, signalling pathways in cancer therapy. *Nat Rev Cancer.* 2003;3(1):11–22.

[9] Katz M, Amit I, Yarden Y. Regulation of MAPKs by growth factors and receptor tyrosine kinases. *Biochim Biophys Acta.* 2007;1773(8):1161–76.

[10] Galabova-Kovacs G, Matzen D, Piazzolla D et al. Essential role of B-Raf in ERK activation during extraembryonic development. *Proc Natl Acad Sci USA* 2006.

[11] Anforth RM, Blumetti TC, Kefford RF, Sharma R, Scolyer RA, Kossard S, et al. Cutaneous manifestations of dabrafenib (GSK2118436): a selective inhibitor of mutant BRAF in patients with metastatic melanoma. *Br J Dermatol.* 2012;167(5):1153–60.103: 1325–1330.

[12] Balagula Y, Lacouture ME, Cotliar JA. Dermatologic toxicities of targeted anticancer therapies. *J Support Oncol* 2010; 8: 149–161.

[13] Peric M, Koglin S, Dombrowski Y et al. VDR and MEK-ERK dependent induction of the antimicrobial peptide cathelicidin in keratinocytes by lithocholic acid. *Mol Immunol* 2009; 46: 3183–3187.

[14] Deng M, Chen WL, Takatori A et al. A role for the mitogen-activated protein kinase kinase kinase 1 in epithelial wound healing. *Mol Biol Cell* 2006; 17: 3446–3455.

[15] Robert C, Arnault JP, Mateus C. RAF inhibition and induction of cutaneous squamous cell carcinoma. *Curr Opin Oncol* 2011; 23: 177–182.

[16] Lacouture M, Chapman P, Ribas A et al. Presence of frequent underlying RAS mutations in cutaneous squamous cell carcinomas and kerato-acanthomas (cuSCC / KA) that develop in patients during vemurafenib therapy. *J Clin Oncol* 29: 2011 (suppl; abstr 8520).

[17] Su F, Viros A, Milagre C et al. RAS Mutations in Cutaneous Squamous-Cell Carcinomas in Patients Treated with BRAF Inhibitors. *N Engl J Med 2012;* 366: 207–215.

[18] Houben R, Becker JC, Kappel A, et al. Constitutive activation of the Ras-Raf signalling pathway in metastatic melanoma is associated with poor prognosis. *J of Carcinogenesis.* 2004;3(1):6.

[19] Jakob JA, Bassett RL, Ng CS, et al. Clinical characteristics and outcomes associated with BRAF and NRAS mutations in metastatic melanoma. *J Clin Oncol.* 2011;29 Suppl:abstr 8500.

[20] Long GV, Menzies AM, Nagrial AM, et al. Prognostic and clinicopathologic associations of oncogenic BRAF in metastatic melanoma. J Clin Oncol. 2011; 29(10):1239–46.

[21] Karasarides M, Chiloeches A, Hayward R, et al. B-RAF is a therapeutic target in melanoma. *Oncogene*. 2004;23;6292–8.

[22] Chu EY, Wanat KA, Miller CJ, Amaravadi RK, Fecher LA, Brose MS, et al. Diverse cutaneous side effects associated with BRAF inhibitor therapy: A clinicopathologic study. *J Am Acad Dermatol.* 2012;67(6):1265–72.

[23] Robert C, Arnault JP, Mateus C. RAF inhibition and induction of cutaneous squamous cell carcinoma. *Curr Opin Oncol.* 2011;23(2): 177–82.

[24] Dubauskas Z, Kunishige J, Prieto VG, Jonasch E, Hwu P, Tannir NM. Cutaneous squamous cell carcinoma and inflammation of actinic keratoses associated with sorafenib. *Clin Genitourin Cancer.* 2009;7(1):20–3.

[25] Hauschild A, Grob JJ, Demidov LV, Jouary T, Gutzmer R, Millward M, et al. Dabrafenib in BRAF-mutated metastatic mela- noma: a multicentre, open-label, phase 3 randomised controlled trial. *Lancet.* 2012;380(9839):358–65.

[26] Arnault JP, Mateus C, Escudier B, Tomasic G, Wechsler J, Hollville E, et al. Skin tumors induced by sorafenib; paradoxic RAS-RAF pathway activation and oncogenic mutations of HRAS, TP53, and TGFBR1. *Clin Cancer Res.* 2012;18(1):263–72.

[27] Long GV, Trefzer U, Davies MA, Kefford RF, Ascierto PA, Chapman PB, et al. Dabrafenib in patients with Val600Glu or Val600Lys BRAF-mutant melanoma metastatic to the brain (BREAK-MB): a multicentre, open-label, phase 2 trial. Lancet Oncol. 2012;13(11):1087–95.

[28] Chu EY, Wanat KA, Miller CJ, Amaravadi RK, Fecher LA, Brose MS, et al. Diverse cutaneous side effects associated with BRAF inhibitor

therapy: A clinicopathologic study. *J Am Acad Dermatol.* 2012;67(6):1265–72.

[29] Dubauskas Z, Kunishige J, Prieto VG, Jonasch E, Hwu P, Tannir NM. Cutaneous squamous cell carcinoma and inflammation of actinic keratoses associated with sorafenib. *Clin Genitourin Cancer.* 2009;7(1):20–3.

[30] Falchook GS, Long GV, Kurzrock R, Kim KB, Arkenau TH, Brown MP, et al. Dabrafenib in patients with melanoma, untreated brain metastases, and other solid tumours: a phase 1 dose- escalation trial. *Lancet.* 2012;379(9829):1893–901.

[31] Anforth RM, Blumetti TC, Kefford RF, Sharma R, Scolyer RA, Kossard S, et al. Cutaneous manifestations of dabrafenib (GSK2118436): a selective inhibitor of mutant BRAF in patients with metastatic melanoma. *Br J Dermatol.* 2012;167(5):1153–60.

[32] Kong HH, Turner ML. Array of cutaneous adverse effects associ- ated with sorafenib. *J Am Acad Dermatol.* 2009;61(2):360–1.

[33] Robert C, Mateus C, Spatz A, Wechsler J, Escudier B. Dermatologic symptoms associated with the multikinase inhibitor sorafenib. *J Am Acad Dermatol.* 2009;60(2):299–305.

[34] Davies H, Bignell GR, Cox C, et al. Mutations of the BRAF gene in human cancer. *Nature.* 2002;417:949–54.

[35] FDA label: Zelboraf (Vemurafenib). San Francisco, CA: Genetech USA Inc. 2011. http://www.accessdata.fda.gov/drugsatfda_docs/ label/2011 /202429s000lbl.pdf. Accessed 2 Dec 2012.

[36] FDA label: Nexavar (Sorafenib). Wayne, NJ: Bayer Healthcare Pharmaceuticals Inc. 2005. http://www.accessdata.fda.gov/ drugsatfda_ docs/label/2011/021923s011lbl.pdf. Accessed 10 Jan 2013

[37] Escudier B, Eisen T, Stadler WM, Szczylik C, Oudard S, Siebels M, et al. Sorafenib in advanced clear-cell renal-cell carcinoma. *N Engl J Med.* 2007;356(2):125–34.

[38] Llovet JM, Ricci S, Mazzaferro V, Hilgard P, Gane E, Blanc JF, et al. Sorafenib in advanced hepatocellular carcinoma. *N Engl J Med.* 2008;359(4):378–90.

[39] Eisen T, Ahmad T, Flaherty KT, Gore M, Kaye S, Marais R, et al. Sorafenib in advanced melanoma: a Phase II randomised discontinuation trial analysis. *Br J Cancer.* 2006;95(5):581–6.

[40] Wilhelm SM, Adnane L, Newell P, Villanueva A, Llovet JM, Lynch M. Preclinical overview of sorafenib, a multikinase inhibitor that targets

both Raf and VEGF and PDGF receptor tyrosine kinase signaling. *Mol Cancer Ther.* 2008;7(10):3129–40

[41] Platz A, Egyhazi S, Ringborg U, Hansson J. Human cutaneous melanoma: a review of NRAS and BRAF mutation frequencies in relation to histogenic subclass and body site. *Mol Oncol.* 2008;1:395–405

[42] Sosman JA, Kim KB, Schuchter L, Gonzalez R, Pavlick AC, Weber JS, et al. Survival in BRAF V600-mutant ad- vanced melanoma treated with vemurafenib. *N Engl J Med.* 2012;366(8):707–14.

[43] Chapman PB, Hauschild A, Robert C, Haanen JB, Ascierto P, Larkin J, et al. Improved survival with vemurafenib in melanoma with BRAF V600E mutation. *N Engl J Med.* 2011;364(26):2507– 16.

[44] Bracarda S, Ruggeri EM, Monti M, Merlano M, D'Angelo A, Ferrau F, et al. Early detection, prevention and management of cutaneous adverse events due to sorafenib: recommendations from the Sorafenib Working Group. *Crit Rev Oncol Hematol.* 2012;82(3):378–86.

[45] Boyd KP, Vincent B, Andea A, Conry RM, Hughey LC. Nonmalignant cutaneous findings associated with vemurafenib *J Am Acad Dermatol.* 2012;67(6):1375–9.

[46] Maddox JS, Kung EF, Petronic-Rosic V, Sethi A. Cutaneous drug eruptions induced by sorafenib: a case series. *J Drugs Dermatol.* 2008;7(9):891–3.

[47] Long GV, Trefzer U, Davies MA, Kefford RF, Ascierto PA, Chapman PB, et al. Dabrafenib in patients with Val600Glu or Val600Lys BRAF-mutant melanoma metastatic to the brain (BREAK-MB): a multicentre, open-label, phase 2 trial. *Lancet Oncol.* 2012;13(11):1087–95.

[48] Flaherty KT, Puzanov I, Kim KB, Ribas A, McArthur GA, Sosman JA, et al. Inhibition of mutated, activated BRAF in metastatic melanoma. *N Engl J Med.* 2010;363(9):809–19.

[49] Sinha R, Edmonds K, Newton-Bishop JA, Gore ME, Larkin J, Fearfield L. Cutaneous adverse events associated with vemurafenib in patients with metastatic melanoma: practical advice on diagnosis, pre- vention and management of the main treatment-related skin toxicities. *Br J Dermatol.* 2012;167(5):987–94.

[50] Boyd KP, Vincent B, Andea A, Conry RM, Hughey LC. Nonmalignant cutaneous findings associated with vemurafenib use in patients with metastatic melanoma. *J Am Acad Dermatol.* 2012;67(6):1375–9.

[51] Scandurra G, Aiello RA, Ali M, Taibi E, Sano MV, Todaro FM, et al. Appropriate management of cutaneous adverse events maxi- mizes

compliance with sorafenib treatment: a single-center expe- rience. *Future Oncol.* 2012;8(5):609–15.

[52] Dummer R, Rinderknecht J, Goldinger SM. Ultraviolet A and photosensitivity during vemurafenib therapy. *N Engl J Med.* 2012;366(5):480–1.

[53] Chu D, Lacouture ME, Fillos T, Wu S. Risk of hand-foot skin reaction with sorafenib: a systematic review and meta-analysis. *Acta Oncol.* 2008;47(2):176–86.

[54] Anderson R, Jatoi A, Robert C, Wood LS, Keating KN, Lacouture ME. Search for evidence-based approaches for the prevention and palliation of hand-foot skin reaction (HFSR) caused by the multikinase inhibitors (MKIs). *Oncologist.* 2009;14(3):291–302.

[55] Bennani-Lahlou M, Mateus C, Escudier B, Massard C, Soria JC, Spatz A, et al. Eruptive nevi associated with sorafenib treatment. *Ann Dermatol Venereol.* 2008;135(10):672–4.

[56] Kong HH, Sibaud V, Chanco Turner ML, Fojo T, Hornyak TJ, Chevreau C. Sorafenib-induced eruptive melanocytic lesions. *Arch Dermatol.* 2008;144(6):820–2.

In: New Skin Toxicities ...
Editors: Giulia Ganzetti et al.
ISBN: 978-1-63482-224-4

Chapter 5

Addendum: Classification of EGFR-Related Skin Rash

K. Giuliodori*[*], *MD, and A. Offidani, MD, Professor
Dermatology Unit, Department of Clinical and Molecular Sciences,
Polytechnic Marche University, Italy

For the definition of toxicity in cancer patients receiving chemotherapy / radiotherapy, a special assessment scale has been established by the National Cancer Institute (NCI) and indicated by the acronym NCI-CTCAE (Common Terminology Criteria National Cancer Institute for Adverse Events) used for reporting adverse events. The latest versions are the NCI-CTCAE v.3 (Table 1) from the year 2006 and NCI-CTCAE v.4 (Table 2) proposed in 2009.

Any adverse event is described through a severity scale including 5 severity degrees: grade 1 (mild), grade 2 (moderate), grade 3 (severe), grade 4 (if the sign/symptom represents a threat to the life or determines disability) and grade 5 (if the adverse event appears to be the cause of death of the patient in treatment).

This evaluation scale has nevertheless proven to be unsuitable and unable to accurately describe dermatological adverse events and in particular the papulopustular rash. It should be stressed that this is an evaluation system designed to define the toxicity secondary to the use of traditional chemotherapy or radiotherapy, and therefore unable to best describe the events

[*] Correspondence to: katiagiuliodori79@yahoo.it.

related adverse to new targeted therapies. Hence the need to propose and develop new grading able to outline and describe more fully the adverse events related EGFR-Is. In this regard, version NCI-CTCAE v.4 updated in 2009 has been introduced, but, however, for dermatologists, it is still not suitable for assessing the severity of the skin lesions and especially to monitor their evolution over time.[1]

Table 1. Classification of acneiform eruption in the course of cancer treatment according to NCI-CTCAE v.3

Grade	Definition
Grade 1	Macular or papular eruption or erythema without associated symptoms
Grade 2	Macular or papular eruption or erythema with pruritus or other associated symptoms; localized desquamation or other lesions covering <50% of body surface area (BSA)
Grade 3	Severe, generalized erythroderma or macular, papular or vescicular eruption; desquamation covering ≥50% BSA
Grade 4	Generalized exfoliative, ulcerative, or bullous dermatitis
Grade 5	Death

Table 2. Classification of acneiform eruption in course of cancer therapy according to NCI-CTCAE v.4

Grade	Definition
Grade 1	Papules and/or pustules covering <10% BSA, which may or may not be associated with symptoms of pruritus or tenderness
Grade 2	Papules and/or pustules covering 10 - 30% BSA, which may or may not be associated with symptoms of pruritus or tenderness; associated with psychosocial impact; limiting instrumental ADL
Grade 3	Papules and/or pustules covering >30% BSA, which may or may not be associated with symptoms of pruritus or tenderness; limiting self care ADL; associated with local superinfection with oral antibiotics indicated
Grade 4	Papules and/or pustules covering any % BSA, which may or may not be associated with symptoms of pruritus or tenderness and are associated with extensive superinfection with IV antibiotics indicated; life-threatening consequences
Grade 5	Death

The grading system proposed by Wollenberg et al. in 2008, the EGFR-index is a score evaluation that defines the severity of the eruption taking into account several parameters and in particular the proportion of involved body and facial skin surface, the presence and distribution of the erythema, presence of papules, pustules and crusts/scales. Using the equation below you get a score based on which it is possible to distinguish the papulo-pustular eruption mild (total score 0-20), moderate (score 21-40 total) or severe (total score 41-100).

EGFR-Index

EGFR index: ¼ A+¼B+ 10/3 (C)
A: Body involvement (0-100%)
B: Facial involvement (0-100%)
C: Skin lesion score: sum of

1. erythema intensity
(none = 0, pale red = 1, moderate = 2, dark red = 3)
2. erythema distribution
(none = 0, scattered = 1, intermediate = 2, dense = 3)
3. papulation (0-3)
4. postulation (0-3)
5. scaling/crusts (0-3)

Eruption

(a) Mild (final score 0-20)
(b) Moderate (final score 21–40)
(c) Severe (final score 41-100).

From the literature it appears evident the need to create a standardized rating scale but especially specific for the definition of the toxicity induced by targeted therapies described. An attempt in this direction was made by MASCC (Multinational Association of Supportive Care in Cancer) Skin Toxicity Study Group that has proposed a new classification method designed specifically for toxicity from EGFR-Is, waiting to be validated [2].

References

[1] National Cancer Institute. Common Terminology Criteria Adverse Events v4.0. *NCI, NHI, DHHS.* May, 29, 2009 NHI publication.

[2] Wollenberg A, Moosmann N, Klein E, Katzer K. A tool for scoring of acneiform skin eruptions induced by EGF receptor inhibition. *Exp Dermatol* 2008;17(9):790-2.

Index

A

B

I

J

K

L

M

N

O

P

Q

R

S